Healing Ceremonies

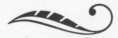

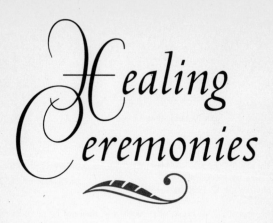

Healing Ceremonies

Creating Personal Rituals
for Spiritual, Emotional,
Physical and
Mental Health

Carl A. Hammerschlag, M.D.

AND

Howard D. Silverman, M.D.

A PERIGEE BOOK

A Perigee Book
Published by The Berkley Publishing Group
200 Madison Avenue
New York, NY 10016

First edition: June 1997

Trade edition ISBN: 0-399-52303-0
Hardcover edition ISBN: 0-399-52358-8

Published simultaneously in Canada.

The Putnam Berkley World Wide Web site address is
http://www.berkley.com

Library of Congress Cataloging-in-Publication Data

Hammerschlag, Carl A.
    Healing ceremonies : creating personal rituals for spiritual,
emotional, physical and mental health / Carl Hammerschlag and
Howard D. Silverman.—1st ed.
        p.   cm.
    "A Perigee book."
    Includes bibliographical references.
    ISBN 0-399-52303-0
    1. Medicine and psychology.   2. Rites and ceremonies—Therapeutic
use.   3. Ritual—Therapeutic use.   4. Healing—Psychological
aspects.   5. Indians of North America—Medicine.   6. Spiritual
healing.   7. Self-care, Health.   I. Silverman, Howard D.
II. Title.
R726.5.H329   1997
615.5—dc21   96-46201
                                                              CIP

Printed in the United States of America

10   9   8   7   6   5   4   3   2   1

For:

My Tushy Princess,
the Red Boy and Ace Baby...

...my conduits to immortality.

—CAH

and

For:

All those who came before me,
who handed these gifts to me
to use with integrity
and pass along.

—HDS

Contents

Contents

ACKNOWLEDGMENTS

To all our relations

To Sharona Silverman, whose presence is between the letters on these pages.

To Sheila Curry and Carol Sowell, whose editorial skills enliven these pages.

To our colleagues, Bernie Siegel, Larry Dossey, Andy Weil, Joan Borysenko and all the other medicine men and women who have also walked this journey.

To our patients, to our students big and small, esteemed teachers and ancestors who kept the flames burning and to storytellers, shamans and mystics everywhere.

And to these friends and relatives: Omer Reed, Judy Hammerschlag, Gershon Winkler, Bill Berk, Mitch Akin, Jonathan Omer-Man, Zalman Schachter-Shalomi, Bill and Vera Tyner, Nelson Fernandez, Christy Stice, Molly Mudick, Thomas Reifers, Joyce Clark and Richard Keelor.

—CAH & HDS

and to

Lisa Jann who organizes my life, Kyle Porter who manages it and Marcia Hancock who records it.

John Koriath, Mona Polacca, Joyce Mills, Dallas Delowe, Harrington and Andrea Luna, Charlesetta Sutton, Tom Howard, Jack Vaughn and all my brothers and sisters in the Turtle Island Project.

And as always, to my children, and always to my love.

—CAH

and to

My Sharona, whose love lifts me up when I fall. And to my daughters, Rachel and Arielle, for being the joy of my life.

My parents, Ina and Dave, for their raising me onto their shoulders.

The Schneiders of Bainbridge Island, whose love is felt afar and especially for Toby, who has always understood me.

All residents and faculty whom I have enjoyed being with both while awake and asleep.

—HDS

Mi Takuye Oyacin

PREFACE

"I will not be for them like a donkey, eternally hauling their books.
I will explain their teachings and study their ways,
but when my vision does not correspond with theirs,
I will then decide according to what my own eyes behold,
and with legal certainty.
For God grants wisdom in every generation and in every period, and
will not deny goodness to those who are sincere."

—Rabbi Moshe ben Nachman, 12th-century Spain
(Introduction to Sefer HaMitzvot L'HaRamban)

Once upon a time . . .

About fifteen years ago we began a most unusual and interesting relationship. Through the years, we have shared the ups and downs of our lives as student and teacher, mentor and student, and now as colleagues. Our relationship has been one of struggle and growth, and our connection has grown stronger because of each experience. We have ensured our relationship's survival because we share a rich ceremonial life together. Ceremonies have helped us to find our way back to the core values of respect, tolerance, and love on which our connection is based.

We invite you to join us in this ceremonial space-time as we tell our stories about what happened "once upon a time."

CARL: *I have already chronicled my coming to Indian country a young, arrogant, New York-born physician-psychiatrist who, for his military obligation, chose to work with the Pueblo tribes of the Southwest. There began an odyssey that took me from doctor to healer.[1]*

For many years, I was the chief of psychiatry at the Phoenix

Indian Medical Center. During that time, I also served on the faculty of several area teaching hospitals with psychiatric residency programs. A young family-practice resident called me one day. He was struggling with his identity in medicine. When he came to the first appointment, he was carrying some insurance forms and told me he'd pay for whatever his insurance didn't cover. I appreciated his telling me that he didn't expect to get something for nothing. But he didn't yet know that money is not the only medium of exchange. Freud knew it; medicine men have always known it—for healing to take place, something of value has to be exchanged between participants. Whether through money, produce, or pieces of art, it is the exchange that gives power. So, I put the papers on my desk and listened to Howie tell his story:

HOWARD: *Even before I had applied to medical school, I watched the way medical school turned people into doctors. I knew physicians in training were sleep-deprived, received constant criticism from instructors, were separated from family and friends, felt their personalities being ground down to conform to a standard. But I thought I could withstand these pressures, and for a long time I did. I learned to look at these trials as one of those periods that all healers go through when they try to deepen their healing abilities. By the time of my residency, though, I started to worry that maybe I was losing it. Despite my determination to stay emotionally close to my patients, I was distancing myself more and more from them. Even more disturbing, I was distancing myself from my family. I was spending so much time wearing the white coat and responding to job demands that I was paying less attention to things that used to give me joy. Some part of me, some part deep inside, was broadcasting a distress signal.*

I knew Carl had been through the medical training process, but he didn't seem to be hard-wired to it. I'd heard he'd worked with Native Americans and spent time singing with them, even going to spiritual gatherings. I hoped he wouldn't look at me in a standard psychiatric way.

I told Carl how detached I was feeling, that I wanted to touch people with my heart, not just with my scientific tools. I needed more contact, more time with people I was treating. But "reality" told me that time was not a reimbursable commodity . . . I had to see more patients . . . it's in the number of patients seen that you make a living, not in the number of patients you touch.

At the end of our first meeting, Carl leaned over his desk and tore up the insurance forms. My first thought was: He doesn't want to see me any more; maybe he's not interested or he can't help me. Then he said, "You're not crazy—let's get together for coffee from time to time and maybe you can arrange to come with me to the reservation some day."

I took my psychiatric rotation with Carl, and the first week he took me to the Hopi reservation. On our small plane were an elderly couple whom he called Sigee (much later, I learned this means "uncle" in Kiowa) and Aunt Vera. I didn't know it then, but I was sitting next to a Pawnee medicine man, a spiritual leader, a healer.

On the way home, the old medicine man invited me to join him in a sweat. I didn't know what it meant, and Sigee (whose name was Bill Tyner) added that he'd like me to check his blood pressure in the sweat lodge. He was making it easy for me to come, and I wanted to go. Wasn't this what I said I was looking for?

He told me a little about the ceremony—that it was a place that helped to make you healthy. The lava rocks that bring in the heat are actually our grandfathers, and their breath is the steam that is created when the rocks are splashed with water. The steam helps you see through your fear and makes you strong.

I picked him up on the following Saturday night, and he took me to a home on the reservation. Outside, a large campfire burned in front of an igloo-shaped willow frame that would later be covered with canvas to form the sweat lodge. Bill invited me into the home and introduced me to the hosts as his personal physician, and I theatrically took his blood pressure on the kitchen table, smiling and going with the program. Afterwards, we joined the men outside who were singing and drumming. When we went into the sweat lodge, the old man introduced me and said he met me in an airplane. He told the men that I see Indian patients and wanted to learn something about healing. When my turn came to speak, I said I appreciated being there and that I wanted to heal myself and to learn as many ways as I could to come to my patients and make a difference to them.

The ceremony was beautiful. I was moved by the prayers which these "relatives" offered for me and my family, for my health and strength, for wisdom. I didn't even know these people, but they prayed that I might bring healing to those who come to me, especially members of their tribe whom I would treat.

As I drove home afterwards, I knew I had turned a corner. That sweat lodge ceremony had helped drain me of some of my fear and rigidity, the instructions and attitudes I'd been accumulating like a side effect of my medical training: Don't introduce yourself by your first name, and maintain an objective, detached, impersonal relationship. That ceremony fanned the spark that had very nearly become extinguished—my connection to the power to heal with joy.

Our relationship has grown over the years, from that of mentor-student to that of colleagues. For fifteen years, we have created and shared rich ceremonial times. These experiences have helped us to grow and to make sense of the events in our lives, and to strengthen our ability to bring forth the gifts our patients need. We have, along with other doctors, nurses, therapists, and people seeking help, discovered that rituals and ceremonies provide the structure that helps us deal with the expected and unexpected transitions in our lives. Rituals and ceremonies help orient us during crises. They facilitate connections, helping us to reframe our experience in more functional ways.

I

About Ceremonies

"Patients carry their own doctor inside.
They come to us not knowing that truth.
We are at our best when we give the physician
who resides within each patient
a chance to go to work."
—Albert Schweitzer

WHAT DO WE MEAN
BY RITUALS AND CEREMONIES?

THE WORDS "RITUAL" and "ceremony" are so widely used that they mean many things to different people. Generally, both words refer to processes that separate the ordinary from the extraordinary. Some of these processes are repetitive (we'll call these rituals) and others may be performed only on special occasions (we'll call these ceremonies).

We all perform "rituals" in our everyday behavior. Think about your typical daily routine. What activities do you repeat "religiously" every day? Do you brush your teeth before you wash your face (or vice versa)? What about your morning coffee, food preparation, driving to work or shopping? What is going on in your mind when you engage in these activities? Most people perform these activities "automatically," with little conscious thought. And how many times have you found yourself thinking about something completely different while you are in the midst of these personal rituals—"daydreaming"? These activities have some of the flavor of ritual or ceremony, in that we temporarily suspend our way of processing data and get into a rhythm in which we do things we seldom overtly think about.

This is a simple example of how we separate the ordinary from the extraordinary. The steps of rituals, repeated every day, are "ordinary" experiences. But our thoughts, daydreams, and associations, which occur at the same time but are unrelated to the ordinary steps of the ritual activity, are "extraordinary." Even a standard morning coffee break is a time to suspend ourselves from the ordinary pressures of the day. You can come to this ordinary daily ritual with an awareness of its ordinary potential and let your mind wander for a few minutes, unruffled by the world around you. Taste the coffee, smell it, get into the moment.

In this book, we use the word "ceremonies" to refer to activities that take place only on special occasions and that are consciously designed to produce beneficial effects. By "rituals" we mean habits we do automatically and without the conscious design and power of ceremonies.

WHAT HAPPENS DURING A CEREMONY?

First, you set aside a special time, where you can slow down and get away from interruptions so you can pay attention. It's a time in which people expect something special is going to happen. Then you find or create a special place—a place that calls to you, that fills you with awe. You can set up a special space by having everybody sit in a circle, or lighting some candles. Add to this a special ceremony (written, spoken, acted, danced, prayed, sung) that someone has created for this moment.

Most of us want to be involved in such happenings because they bring us closer to ourselves and to each other in a special way. We need to get together more often in ceremonial time and space because ceremonies provide the opportunity to reframe, reinvent and retell the stories that help us make sense of our lives. It is through the telling and sharing of stories that we share our most fundamental truths from one heart to the next.

Telling stories in ceremonies helps us to listen better and provide a lens through which we can see things in a new light. They provide the structure by which we can lift our hearts from self-doubt. They provide access into the world of faith and the human spirit. Ceremonies help provide road maps that restore our dreams, express our visions, and give us hope. They provide us with a time to experience awe—a state in which we lift ourselves out of the ordinary into a different level of consciousness. Awe is the ultimate reminder that we are small and the universe is large. Awe helps us to find the faith to move forward. In fact, much has been gained through "leaps of faith" that could not have been achieved by certainty or planning.

Rabbi Lawrence Kushner describes awesome, yet fleeting moments that often coincide with religious ceremonies marking life's passages, such as Bar or Bat Mitzvah, a wedding, or a funeral. At such times, he says, "We realize that we are part of something much larger than our daily decisions. With or without our consent, we too are players in a kind of divine scheme. Of course, it is preposterous, and it makes no rational sense, but for just a moment or two it is as if we rise to encounter our destiny: It was not you who sent me here, but God!"[2]

People in every religion and every culture have used ceremonies and rituals to help make sense out of the experiences of their lives and to teach ethical ways of breathing meaning into life. In order to touch and be touched in healing ways, you must be connected to a belief in something bigger than yourself. Whatever that belief is, from God to astrology, old-growth forests or the family homeland, during ceremonial time you experience your life as an unfolding drama whose meaning is broader than day-to-day concerns. Ceremony is a time to seek guidance, to share in community, to look within, to touch people, practices, dreams, and imagination. Ceremonies can help provide a way to get in touch with courage and inspiration in order to find healing in symbolic form.

In modern societies, the role of ceremony has become narrowly defined and its expression constrained. Because we have invested science with providing all the answers, we've come to believe that the secrets of life can be known only through proven quantitative means. We have thus come to master the natural processes and create better living conditions. As a result, we have also created a culture in which we subordinate the subjective experience of our lives to objective reality, even though that "objectivity" flows from fact fragments based on somebody else's perception of what's probable. In doing so, we give up our dreams, and we surrender our possibilities to their probabilities. Without dreams, we can become only what we see now and can never achieve what we dare to imagine.

All too often the ceremonies that are available to us have lost their inner meaning. Think about how modern commercialism has squeezed virtually all spiritual meaning out of the celebrations of Christmas and Thanksgiving. While the core meanings of these holidays are still celebrated by some, most people associate them only with "having to" buy gifts, hours of work in the kitchen, and "getting through" a shared experience with relatives. We are in danger of desacralizing the sacred.

There is a company that sells the wine and bread of Holy Communion in prepackaged cups. The all-in-one cups (which look like containers of coffee creamers) are passed out to congregants. One pastor said, "It's just very convenient to use, cuts the distribution time at least in half."

The sacred has been mass-marketed at the expense of true spirituality. In a society that worships speed and convenience over belief in miracles, we tend to isolate ourselves more and more from our spirit. It makes the sacred seem awfully sterile.

WHY ARE CEREMONIES IMPORTANT?

Ceremonies helped our ancestors live rich lives. As life has sped up over the centuries, we have become increasingly less tolerant of things that take time. When we no longer listen to those who tell the stories that speak of eternal values, who help us to center our lives, then we become consumed by immediate gratification and personal power. In cultures where product overshadows process, we undervalue, even ignore, the importance of a ritual life. When the moments of our lives are less valued than the material, we stifle our vital forces and become susceptible to disease.

How can we tap into the sustaining dimension that can help us make sense of the events in our lives and even get us through them? Rituals and ceremonies can provide the vehicle for reshaping what we say and feel, and how we express ourselves. Participating in ceremonies such as weddings, coming-of-age celebrations, funerals, and observations of solstices can influence our beliefs and behaviors, and reconnect us with our spiritual selves.

What is the spiritual self? It's not easy to define in scientific terms, nor is it necessary to do so. The spiritual self is that quality of human beings that can be felt but not touched, perceived but not seen. Lao-tzu, a legendary Chinese philosopher who lived five hundred years before the birth of Christ, suggested that truth, wisdom, goodness, beauty, and the fragrance of a rose are all linked spiritually in that they are intangible, ineffable realities. The distinguished physician Deepak Chopra echoes the awe of the paradoxes of spirit, noting that "The spirit is a real force. It's as real as gravity, it's as real as time. It's equally abstract, equally as incomprehensible and mysterious and difficult to grasp conceptually. It's very powerful, and when we touch that spiritual core of awareness, only then can we be healed."[3]

We believe that true healing requires the participation of one's spiritual self. We believe that stories and ceremonies are the surest ways of touching the human spirit and promoting healing. When it comes to healing, how we feel is at least as important as what we know. This is true for both patient and healer because both must connect with feeling if they are to maximize their shared healing journey. Carl Jung, the visionary psychoanalyst, wrote, "We should not pretend to understand the world only by the intellect; we apprehend it just as much by feeling. Therefore the judgment of the intellect is, at best, only the half of truth, and must, if it be honest, also come to an understanding of its inadequacy."[4]

As a species, what we feel has evolved little over the last 100,000 years. We experience the same fears, disasters, and mysteries that ancient people faced, although we also may have engineered different modes of disaster and disease such as airplane crashes and heart disease. The ancient ones learned some things that we ought to pay attention to. They knew that staying well was only a means to an end. In most ancient cultures, the ultimate goal was spiritual maturation, a transcendental experience, something that elevated the human spirit. They were certain that survival meant sustaining the mystical fire. Appreciating mystery and awe is what ultimately helps us make sense of our lives and play our part in the greater universe. Albert Einstein, our century's foremost scientific genius, understood this perfectly when he said, "The most beautiful and profound emotion we can ever experience is the mystical."

CEREMONY AND MODERN MEDICINE

Getting sick has at least as much to do with how you come to the germ emotionally as it does with how the germ physically comes to you.[5]

Today, medicine stands at a crossroads. It is becoming increasingly clear that the tremendous advances of science are costly both financially and physically. While the financial cost is generating increasing concern in industry and government, the cost of traditional medicine denying the underlying issues of meaning and spirit in health is distressing to our patients. One marker for this trend is the high level of use of "alternative medicine" practitioners in the United States. One recent study found that 34 percent of respondents reported using at least one unconventional therapy in the past year. The most common types of therapies were self-help groups, acupuncture, megavitamin therapy, massage, and relaxation techniques, costing approximately $13.7 billion, three-quarters of which ($10.3 billion) was paid out of pocket.[6] On the one hand, this level of interest may lead to more studies of these practices. But while some provide spiritual and physical healing, the potential for hucksterism and health hoaxes remains worrisome. In an attempt to bring a spiritual or nonmedical approach to healing, people may actually be putting their health in jeopardy.

One of our goals in writing this book is to convey that medicine and spirit are not incompatible. Rather, combining one with the other creates potential for healing that goes far beyond the potential of either one used independently. Some doctors may say that what we're advocating sounds suspiciously like witchcraft or wishful thinking, but we've both successfully used ceremony as a practical method to integrate science and spirit.

Consider Howard's wife, Sharona's, experiences:

I had been experiencing the increasing disfigurement of scoliosis, a curvature of the spine. Ultimately, I decided the risks of corrective surgery were less than the complications of allowing the disease to progress. A surgeon installed metal hardware along my spine from the middle of my rib cage to the base of my spine. About a week after surgery, a friend volunteered to come by my hospital room and wash my hair. My husband happened to be there when she arrived, and he agreed to be her assistant. She lovingly washed my hair as my husband carried warm water in a small hospital pitcher back and forth to the bedside. My thoughts turned to the biblical stories of Abraham washing the feet of visiting strangers.

Without prompting, my husband was moved to light some ceremonial sweetgrass, a Native American purification ritual that we sometimes use. We played some tapes that were very special to me. The three of us worked in unison without saying one word.

Suddenly there was a knock at the door and my orthopedic surgeon entered. He strode confidently toward the bed and then abruptly stopped, as if he had just hit an invisible wall. He observed us for a moment, the silence, the washing, the music, the sweet smell. He smiled and said, "I don't want to disturb you. I'll see you tomorrow." We thanked him and he left. What a gift of insight to recognize that what we were doing had importance to us, even if he chose not to participate. Imagine the healing effect if he had stayed for a few moments and offered to carry a pitcher of warm water!

In this spontaneous ceremony, with sweetgrass, music, and warm water as its sacraments, Sharona's orthopedist could have magnified his healing power if he'd understood that the ceremony was a way of welcoming her back to the world. In addition to his surgical skills, he could have connected at the level of heart and spirit, further helping her to heal.

Modern medical culture separates patients from their physicians. That separation can never result in true healing. True healing only occurs when both participants are connected in pursuing the common goal of healing. This connection promotes healing and should be expressed in every form available. This partnership also works both ways and affords the physician with the opportunity to grow and to become reenergized. A colleague of Howard's related the following:

Once I started asking my patients about their spiritual lives, a whole new world opened up before me. Many of my patients were eager to share their spiritual concerns with me. What I discovered, to my delight and surprise, was that I became increasingly energized by these connections. In spite of my heavy workload in the office, I found myself being more and more excited about coming in each morning, looking forward to being with my patients in a new way—a way which allowed both of us to grow together.

While we are ceremonialists, we also honor our origins as scientists. As the field of psychoneuroimmunology (PNI) unfolds, it offers some highly interesting evidence that helps explain our empiric observations of ceremonies at work. This new science is predicated on the assumption that beliefs, feelings, and the functioning of our immune systems are intimately linked. Laboratory research is now documenting what healers have long known anecdotally. How we feel is connected to what we believe, and this is true for both patient and healer. When it comes to participating fully in our own health, how we feel is probably more important.

PNI emphasizes a view of the body as an integrated circuit. In health, the brain, the blood, the glands, and the nerves all work cooperatively to guard against disease. They work together through constant communication to mobilize and modulate each other's power in combating disease and maintaining balance. These influences can express themselves both positively and negatively. If you stay depressed, you'll also depress your immune system; conversely, if you feel good and can harness your body's power, you strengthen your immune response.

Several excellent PNI reviews are available, ranging from the highly scientific[7,8,9,10,11,12] to those written more for the lay reader.[13,14,15] They describe two principal links that join science and ceremonies. The first is connection and the second is the telling of the story. Those are the means through which rituals and ceremonies help orient us during crises. Through connection and stories, rituals link us with people who make a difference in our lives. Rituals and ceremonies provide credible connections that help us get through trials.

FEELING CONNECTED

How can simply feeling more connected with ourselves and with other people lead to better health? While the exact mechanisms are still not entirely clear, there is evidence to support this contention.

Women with cancer who participate in support groups live longer than those without such groups; divorced and widowed people (especially men) in their twenties and thirties have a much higher risk of dying than married persons of the same age; marital conflict has negative effects on the immune system; there's a link between the death of a spouse and impairment of the immune function; social isolation is a major risk factor for mortality from widely varying causes. It has been found that social support mitigates the harmful effects of stressful life events.

Several investigations have attempted to clarify the link between social support and a lower risk of cardiovascular disease. One study of patients in a coronary care unit showed that being connected to other people has a beneficial effect even when the recipient is not aware of the connection. In this analysis, heart patients were assigned randomly to two groups. The control group of patients had no intervention, while the names of the patients in the treatment group were given to individuals who prayed for them, but without any actual contact with the patient. The authors noted that "the control patients required ventilatory assistance, antibiotics, and diuretics more frequently than patients in the intercessory prayer group."[16]

Science has begun to notice something that healers have always known: Feeling connected to people and things outside yourself helps to keep you healthy and assists you when you're ill. Even, as in the above example, when the patients themselves were unaware that a connection had been forged!

THE TELLING OF THE STORY

The second connection between PNI and ceremonies is the telling of the story. We all have a set of stories or myths by which we explain the world and our place in it. We are given these stories early in life by those whose function is to help orient us toward living in the world. When change occurs, some of us hang on to the old stories that once made sense to us, but that have become dysfunctional in a new environment. Some stories, on the other hand, help us to confront life's changes and difficulties. To keep healthy, we have to look at whether our personal, cultural, and religious stories are working for us. If they aren't, we need to rewrite them.

Negative or dysfunctional stories learned in childhood can cause problems later in life if they are not somehow changed. Chronic negativity or pessimism directed at a child is a predictor of depressive symptoms later in life.[17] Your view of the world can also predict immune system dysfunction. Researchers studying elderly men and women have found that "a pessimistic style might be an important psychological risk factor (at least among older people) in the early course of certain immune-mediated diseases."[18] Such diseases include cancer, asthma, infections, and arthritis.

Writing and telling a new story is a powerful way of taking control over life's challenges and exercising your options. Being able to make choices in your life creates an atmosphere, both emotionally and at a cellular level, that promotes health. Conversely, when you believe yourself to be powerless in determining your destiny, you fail to thrive. One example of this is data showing that people in old age homes live longer when they have a choice about what to eat, furniture arrangement, plants, or pets.[19,20]

Choice makes a difference, even to animals. A rat injected with cancerous cells and then presented with an inescapable electric shock every few minutes will die from the complications of the cancer much more quickly than an identical twin that is taught to escape the shocks.[21] Choice is the greatest power you have; it's your right and privilege as an adult. *Believing* you can influence your destiny makes a difference at every level of your being. You have choices even in circumstances in which you seem enslaved.

Viktor Frankl, a remarkable psychiatrist, was imprisoned in the infamous Auschwitz concentration camp.[22] As a physician with a marketable skill, he was not selected for immediate extermination. Instead, he lined up with others who had also been momentarily spared.

After days locked in a cattle car, the prisoners were all starving. The man standing next to Frankl stepped on a grasshopper and bent over to pick it up and eat it. An SS guard, upon seeing him, walked over and beat the starving man to death on the spot.

At that moment, Frankl made a decision that, he said, saved his life. He realized he had no choice over whether his tormentors killed him by beating or gas, by starvation or torture. But he did have this choice: Independent of their decision regarding his life or death, he would not let them rob him of his dignity.

Even as a prisoner, whether of illness, financial problems, or other circumstances, you have the capacity to choose your attitude, to transcend suffering, and to find meaning in life. Choice elevates the spirit by allowing you to exercise your responsibilities to yourself and your faith. Only a fraction of the stories of choice have survived to be told, such as this report by an eyewitness who survived the Nazi concentration camps.

The train dragged on with its human freight. Pressed together like cattle in the crowded trucks, the unfortunate occupants were unable even to move. The atmosphere was stifling. As the Friday afternoon wore on, the Jewish men and women in the Nazi transport sank deeper and deeper into their misery.

Suddenly an old Jewish woman managed with a great effort to move and open her bundle. Laboriously she drew out two candlesticks and two challoth (traditional Sabbath bread). She had prepared them for Sabbath when she was dragged from her home that morning. They were the only things she had thought worth taking with her. Soon the Sabbath candles lit up the faces of the tortured Jews and the songs of the Sabbath transformed the scene. Sabbath with its atmosphere of peace had descended upon them all.[23]

Another dramatic example of this phenomenon of choice is the story of a blind man named Jacques Lusseyran. In his autobiography, he described how the "gift" of blindness was a source of unique happiness for him. He chose, despite his disability, to meet any challenge with joy, love, and what he called the "light within." Lusseyran was active in the French resistance during World War II. After being caught by the Gestapo, he spent fifteen months in the Buchenwald concentration camp. Of the two thousand Frenchmen who were shipped to this camp along with Lusseyran, only thirty were alive at the end of the war. He recalled that, with death present every moment, he was able to choose to retreat to the inner light within. He explained, "Our fate is shaped from within ourselves outward, never from without inward."[24]

No matter how bad things get, you can choose to create your story in a new and healthier way.

We believe that ceremonies have the potential to strengthen the body's immune response.[25,26] Contemporary medical training does not teach its practitioners how to connect ceremonially with an open heart. Instead, we are trained to believe that to see clearly means to control and even deny our own feelings. We are taught that sharing ourselves will distort our clinical objectivity: Don't get too close to your patients. Perhaps this is why physicians as a group are not altogether healthy. Long hours and unremitting exposure to the tragedies of life can wear down anybody's body and soul. Studies have indicated that physicians commit suicide at a rate four times higher than the general population.[27,28,29] For physicians over age 65, this rate jumps to nearly fifteen times that of the general population. Could this be in part due to the inability of doctors to achieve and maintain balance in their work and their lives? Perhaps the use of ceremonial techniques would allow doctors to be more rounded, refreshed, and balanced human beings and this would, in some way, reduce the despair and frustration reflected in these alarming suicide statistics.

This is how a Native American healer told Carl a story that beautifully illustrates the importance of the health of the healer.

I once asked a 93-year-old Mayan medicine man, Don Eligio, who is considered a national treasure in his country, what was the most important thing he'd learned that enabled him to heal. He answered: "Don't take a cold drink on an empty stomach on a hot day." I looked at him dumbfounded. I asked the interpreter to repeat the question. The medicine man repeated, looking at me, laughing and shaking his head, "The most important thing I've learned to be able to heal people was not to take a cold drink on an empty stomach on a hot day."

I laughed and asked him what it meant.

He said, "It gives you bad belly."

"Bad belly?"

He replied, "With a bad belly, you can't heal."

It took me a little while to understand the wisdom of his answer.

As doctors, most of us come to our patients with well-trained heads and poorly trained "bellies" (or hearts). We are even taught that our power is enhanced if we come with no "belly" at all. We understand the technology, but we ignore the spirit of healing. At age 93, Don Eligio knew with certainty that the most important ingredient in being a healer is to come to your patients with "good belly."

SOME WARNINGS

We are not suggesting that ceremonies replace other medical treatments. Rather, we are challenging ourselves, our patients, our readers, and our colleagues to become more thoughtful about using all the elements in the healing process.

Having said this, let us add that as we have grown in

experience, it has become apparent that healing is complex and mysterious. Pharmaceuticals, surgery, and incantations all have magical powers. Each has a unique place in the healing mystery and none stands alone. We are all in it together. By sharing skills and spirit we intensify our healing powers.

We've also learned that the ultimate goals of all healing practices are connection and expression. If physical healing occurs along the way (as we believe it often does), it is a blessing. If it does not occur, then so be it. In his recent book, *Healing Words: The Power of Prayer and the Practice of Medicine*, Dr. Larry Dossey beautifully discusses similar issues related to prayer and healing when he states that "Prayerfulness—not the world-manipulating, disease-bashing forms of prayer to which most Westerners resort when sick—permeates many cases of profound illness that improve spontaneously. Prayerfulness allows us to reach a plane of experience where illness can be experienced as a natural part of life, and where its acceptance transcends passivity. If the disease disappears, we are grateful; if it remains, that too is reason for gratitude."[30]

Rabbi Harold Kushner writes about the hope that we can compel God to do as we wish if only we perform the right rituals. "When people assume that because they have been ethically upright and ritually observant, God owes them good health and good fortune, their understanding of what it means to be religious veers dangerously in the direction of magic, doing what religion asks of us not out of love and loyalty, but as a way of controlling God's actions in response."[31]

WHAT IS THIS BOOK ALL ABOUT?

Ceremonies and rituals can be powerful tools in helping us to harness the power to deal with the important transitional events in our lives. When dealing with physical illness, ceremonies can and should serve as *complements* to standard medical diagnostic and therapeutic practices. When examined closely, current medical procedures are revealed to be highly ceremonialized events: the entourage at hospital rounds, the ceremonial instruments used to perform specialized procedures, how office visits are structured. All present different types of ceremonial activities. Imagine how we could maximize our effectiveness if we learned to use them all! One of Howard's patients shared this story with him about a ceremony she had created on her own:

Cindy knew that the blood in her stools was a sign of something terrible happening in her body. Her physician shared her concern and suggested that she undergo a diagnostic test called a barium enema. In this procedure, he explained, special X-ray pictures of her colon would help show the source of the bleeding. Although he didn't mention it specifically, Cindy knew that cancer was one of the possibilities. The nurse gave her a gallon jar of clear liquid and some written directions on how to prepare for the test. She was to drink this fluid before the test in order to clean out the colon and obtain the best possible pictures.

As she drove home from the doctor's office, a million thoughts raced through Cindy's mind, yet she felt surprisingly calm. On an impulse, she stopped and bought an elegant champagne glass and a beautiful bathrobe. When she got home, she unpacked her purchases and placed them on the kitchen table next to the gallon of liquid. "If I must face this, then I will do it my way," she mused. She placed the liquid outdoors in a bed of flowers to absorb the light of the sun and moon for twenty-four hours and then moved it to the refrigerator for storage.

On the morning before the X-ray examination, Cindy put on the robe, turned off the telephone, and spent the day in solitude, sipping the cooled liquid from her new champagne glass. As she did so, she reflected on her life—what was good, what was bad, what needed changing, what needed healing. On the day of the examination, she felt calm, centered, and at peace. She took her special bathrobe to the hospital, and it helped her feel comfortable.

After the exam, the radiologist approached her worriedly and asked her to call her doctor for her test results. "It's cancer, isn't it?" she asked the doctor when he phoned later that day. "Yes, I'm afraid so," he replied, surprised by her composure.

Cindy committed herself to making needed changes in her life and underwent surgery for the colon cancer. Fortunately, the tumor had been detected before it had spread beyond the bowel. She still comes to see me annually for her checkups, and I share with her how I now use her method with other patients.

Cindy's ability to turn a barium enema into a personal ceremony is a powerful lesson. You can approach contemporary diagnostic and therapeutic procedures as if they were an invitation to personal growth rather than something out of a medical textbook. Ceremonializing "routine" medical procedures expands them into events that invite fuller participation in, and responsibility for, the healing process.

This book is meant to help you remember a time in your life when anything was possible, when you had dreams that good things would happen. This book is about recapturing your spirit so you can become the principal agent in your own healing.

The stories in Section II are told in the languages of science and mythology. They show how choice, connectedness, and ceremony influenced the outcome of events in people's lives.

Section III provides some specific approaches to creating healing ceremonies. In some cases, this requires the construction of an altogether new ceremony. In others, you may be able to customize an existing ceremony to better meet your needs. We have included some tips for "ceremonializing" standard medical procedures as well.

In Indian country, to be healthy means to be in balance. Balance occurs when what you know is the same as what you say, and when what you say is how you really feel. Balance happens when knowledge, feeling, and action are in harmony. That is the essence of your being, your truth. The Navajo call this path "Hozho," the way of beauty. To be healthy is to walk in beauty.

When a person is out of harmony with this world, then sickness or misfortune results. Ceremonies are then performed that are intended to restore harmony and thus reverse the potential for danger.

In large part, the ceremonies take the form of chants such as the Nightway Chant. All of them have been given to the Navajo people by representatives of the spirit world. These chants are performed over a period of one, two, three, five or even nine nights. The chants are repetitive and exacting. Each word is essential to ensure the effectiveness of the ceremony.

This is how Navajo medicine men end their Nightway ceremony.

I will walk with a cool body after they have left me.
Inside of me today will be well.
All fever will have come out of me and go away from me and leave
my head cool.
I will hear today.
I will see today.
I will be in my right mind today.
Today I will walk out.
Today everything evil will leave me.
I will be as I was before.
I will have a cool breeze over my body.
I will walk with a light body.
I will be happy forever.
Nothing will hinder me.
I walk in front of me beautiful.
I walk behind me beautiful.
Under me beautiful.
On top of me beautiful.
Around me beautiful.
My words will be beautiful.

I will be everlasting one.
Everything is beautiful.
In beauty may I walk.

This is our wish for you—may you walk in beauty.

II

The Ceremonial Seasons

"Of course it was not I who cured.
It was the power from the outer world,
and the visions and ceremonies had only made me
like a hole through which the power would come to the two-leggeds.
If I thought that I was doing it myself,
the hole would close up and no power would come through it."
—*Black Elk, Oglala Sioux Medicine Man*
(Black Elk Speaks)

DAWN
Childhood (Birth to Age 13)

House made of Dawn
As I awaken to new light
Happily may I walk
Happily with abundant showers may I walk
Happily on the trail of pollen may I walk
Happily may I walk
—from the Navajo Nightway Chant

WHAT IS THE work of infancy? The beginning of life is the season to be nurtured and supported. This is the time to learn to trust. Infants raised with care and love learn to trust that somebody out there will take care of them when they're hurting, feed them when they're hungry, and keep them safe. Through your parents' nurturing, you learn that there's someone who's been waiting for you, someone who loves you and wants you to feel good, who believes you are an important contribution to their world. The work of infancy is being loved and supported and building trust.

This is a Hopi ceremony of awakening which is done to welcome Hopi babies to the world and to their community. The first morning point of light is life reemerging from the underworld. That point is the bellybutton of creation. It is the first breath on the road of life.

For the first twenty days of its life, a Hopi newborn is kept in darkness. On the dawn of the twentieth day the infant is carried to the sacred kiva, the ceremonial heart chamber that is the soul of the Hopi way of life. There, the mother holds her daughter wrapped in a ceremonial blanket and says, "Thank you, Creator, for my daughter. Thank you for this gift of life. I say thank you for all of the gifts of life that you have provided for me. You have created this flesh; you have made the shape of all things. I give my daughter to you to follow in this way."

Jewish males are traditionally welcomed in a similar fashion. On the seventh day of life, before his circumcision, the infant Jewish male is held aloft by his godparent, called the Sandik. If possible, this is a relative of the deceased person for whom the child is named. This person offers a blessing connecting the child to his namesake and to his people. Here is how Carl recalls this special moment:

I ask you, God of the Universe, to bless my grandson, Aaron, who carries the name of my father. Make him a joy to his parents, a holy name among his people and a reflection of your goodness here on Earth. Creator, bless him with the name of my father whose light still shines in my eyes. Bless him, in a good way, on this path of life.

There are many traditional welcome-to-the-world ceremonies. All ways share their wisdom. In each case, the new life is acknowledged and ceremonially connected to the family or tribe. Becoming family means to become part of a community. When the biological bonds to the infant are extended to include familial, communal, and ritual ties, the child grows healthy. Infants draw strength from all those connections who care for them.

As parents, we dream that our children will have the best that life can give. But sometimes the way we wish to know and see our children is not the way they are. They are born different or develop differently from what we imagined and wished for. We must find a way to welcome them as they are, to provide love and allow them to trust, without always feeling our disappointment or judgment. The developmental task for parents is to reconcile the discrepancy between their fantasy of the child and the actual child.[1,2,3] Howard relates the following story about how he and his wife, Sharona, responded to finding out that their newborn daughter, Arielle, was completely blind:

> Sharona realized that Arielle's eyes were not focusing normally when she was two weeks old. After months of difficult visits to doctors, we were told that she was blind. As the weeks passed, Sharona and I had difficulty talking about Arielle's blindness. Both of us were grieving, but not together. Driving home from a summer vacation, we talked about what was happening and we decided to create a ceremony. The purpose was clear to us: We needed to let go of our expectations about this child and to welcome her for who she was and not for what we had hoped she would be.
>
> We consulted our rabbi to see if there was a Jewish Blind Kid ceremony. Not surprisingly, there was none, but he helped us formulate our own. We worked as a team to plan and prepare for the ceremony.

We asked participants to bring to the ceremony their fears and hopes for Arielle, and some food to share afterwards.

I introduced each of the participants and welcomed them using a Native American smudging ceremony that I liked. It is a purification ritual in which herbal smoke is fanned over the body with an eagle feather to ceremonially cleanse whatever ordinary consciousness still clings to the person from the world outside the ceremony.

My wife and I each shared some of our difficult thoughts about Arielle, about our previous expectations for her, our sadness at her lack of sight. Sharona said it would be hard for her to be unable to look into her infant daughter's eyes and bond that way. Then she said, "I know she will remind me of the deeper connections we make with those we love." I mourned that Arielle would never be able to appreciate the visual splendors of nature—she would never be able to see the Grand Canyon, rainbows, clouds, or a sunset. I hoped that, instead, Arielle would teach me to pay more attention to nature's sounds, smells, and textures.

We invited everyone in the circle to share some thoughts, words, or feelings. Each one, with tears and laughter, expressed his or her sorrows and hopes. In speaking about the double pain he felt for his son and for his granddaughter, my father realized why he had avoided holding her. Some people preferred to write down things they were uncomfortable saying out loud, then burned the papers in our fireplace. I sprinkled the burning slips of paper with cedar and sage as our rabbi led us in the recitation of the traditional Jewish mourner's prayer. This ancient prayer declared that we were choosing to let go of the old expectations and to allow a new awareness to be born.

Everyone involved felt a sense of healing and connection. It was as if time had suddenly stood still and we were physically, emotionally, mentally, and spiritually in a place where new stories could be birthed. Even though we had come together for a particular purpose, a friend told me later that the experience had awakened a heightened insight into some issues in her own life.

After the ceremony, Arielle woke up and started crying. My mother tried to comfort her, but couldn't. My father came over and asked to hold her. It was the first time he had come close to her since her birth. He picked her up and she stopped crying instantly. They have been buddies ever since!

The effect of this ceremony was and still is startling. Now, more than ten years later, the potentials we saw have all been realized. The ceremony helped to turn negatives into positives and taught us the true meaning of the phrase "If life gives you lemons, make lemonade."

Now I take walks with Arielle at sunset, and when I close my eyes, I can hear the birds singing everywhere.

This event has all the elements of a healing ceremony. It opens with a welcoming ritual to make everyone a part of the circle. The lighting of sage and fanning it onto each participant brushes off the old clinging dust of yesterday's preconceptions and helps them be truly present in the moment. All those present express themselves about the purpose of this ceremony. They all knew they must adjust their expectations for Arielle, and learn to love her as she is. With symbols and within community, friends and family came together in an event that brought feelings to the surface and invited all involved to unite in the common purpose of healing. This was not an attempt to cure Arielle, but rather to heal the pain of lost expectations. It was also a chance for those who loved Arielle and her family to come together with support and hope for her.

Feelings serve as the language of acceptance or rejection between parents and their infant children. In this ceremony, the parents took a step back, renewed their connection to their newborn daughter, and embraced a new story yet to be written. In doing so, they immediately telegraphed love and acceptance to their daughter. This ceremony addressed the transitional needs of three generations while reintegrating the family's community of friends and relatives to help meet Arielle's special needs.

The power of the ceremony was increased significantly by the addition of ancient Jewish liturgy, including the mourner's prayer (Kaddish). By incorporating this ceremonial element, the group aligned itself with thousands of years of tradition and relatives who have experienced similar thoughts and feelings. Moreover, the spiritual wisdom embodied in this prayer moved the group forward into a new set of possibilities, a new story. The opening and closing of the ceremony, as well as the careful attention paid to the creation and gentle maintenance of boundaries between participants, helped each person feel safe, let go, and be open to new possibilities. These elements heightened trust, which in turn helped the celebrants share the feelings that accompany change: anxiety, excitement, fear, and melancholy.

Here is Barry Neil Kaufman's story:[4]

My wife sensed something was wrong with our newborn son almost from the beginning. In the first month he was crying day and night, he was unresponsive when he was held or fed, but when the doctor examined him he said he was perfectly healthy. When he was a month old he had such a severe ear infection that it ruptured both his ear-

drums. *By the time he was a year old, he was responding less and less to his name and was more profoundly unresponsive. By the time he was seventeen months old, the doctors identified Raun as profoundly intellectually and functionally retarded. They told my wife how terribly sad they were, because the prognosis for this illness is dismal. I thought, "I don't want to look at my son in that way, as terrible and unfortunate," and this was not denial on my part because I knew that my son had been dropped here from another planet and I kept hearing that he would become a severely dysfunctional human being, but my wife looked at Raun and wanted to see something unique, not terrible. We wanted to look at him with wonder, and it was very hard. He developed rampant autistic behavior patterns. He was only happy with himself. He could concentrate on a simple object for hours. At the same time there was something gentle, soft, beautiful about him that we could celebrate as a gift. We decided not to send him away to an institution, which we were told is something we ought to focus on sooner rather than later, and instead we found in him things that happened that opened us up to wonder. We spent a lot of time with him, and there came a time when he could speak a word, although it took him a lot longer and we had to stay on him and focus. But there were other difficult times. We always saw small progress. By the time he was three and a half, he could read first-and second-grade books. We still had to be on him because without energetic stimulation, he would withdraw, but never again into his autistic world.*

Eventually, Raun Kaufman graduated with honors from his high school with his chronological age group and then from an Ivy League university. The Kaufmans used their experience with their son to found the Option Institute in Sheffield, Massachusetts, which has now become an internationally renowned learning center. Families come to the institute with children who face a host of disabilities. They learn how to let go of their judgments and how to use rituals to create new ceremonies to reach out to previously unreachable children.

Ceremony is a way to reconnect with the dreams of our lives, to cleanse ourselves of old expectations, and to make new commitments. It opens us up to being blessed, to new vision, to celebrating joy.

A sadness in contemporary American life is that many children come into the world to people who don't want them, or who are so ill prepared to be parents that their fears overwhelm their love. If you learn in infancy that you are unloved, that your needs will not be met, when you're hungry you won't be fed, when you're dirty you won't be cleaned, when you're hurting you won't be cuddled—then you learn early that this road of life is cruel, hostile, and withholding. Children with this kind of infancy trust no one later in life. If you don't learn to trust that your needs will be met in the early years, then you may never trust or connect with others around you.[5,6]

Beyond infancy and the early developmental years come the struggles of childhood. Even if you are connected with love, things can happen in the flower of youth that pluck the bud before full blossom, as Carl recounts:

In Phoenix, a seven-year-old boy with leukemia had a long period of remission after his initial treatment. After a year, he had a relapse. He was placed on high doses of toxic medications that left him ex-

tremely weak. When his breathing became irregular, the doctors thought he would soon die.

His mother called the Make-A-Wish Foundation, which grants last wishes to dying children. Her son had always wanted to be a fireman, so arrangements were made for him to leave the hospital for a day and visit a Phoenix fire station. The anticipation and fanfare alone were enough to rally him.

At the firehouse, the firefighters took him for a ride through the city streets on a hook and ladder truck with sirens blaring. His face was bright, even though his body was limp. After the ride, they had a special ceremony for him at the firehouse. They gave him a fireman's hat and a jacket with their battalion insignia on it and his name embroidered over the pocket. Every firefighter shook his hand and welcomed him as their newest member. It was the happiest day of his young life.

Back in the hospital, he improved enough to be discharged for several weeks. But when his breathing became gasping and irregular, he was readmitted. Now he was only intermittently conscious. His mother, sensing that the end was near, asked the nurse if her son could see the firemen again. The nurse, who knew how important the visit to the firehouse had been to the boy, agreed to waive the two-visitors-at-a-time requirement.

When the mother called the fire station to ask them to come over, the firemen said, "We'll do better than that. Unlatch the window to his room and tell the nurse to announce over the loudspeaker system that patients should not be alarmed by the sirens. It's just the Fire Department coming to pay respects to one of their own."

Within minutes, the sirens of the approaching hook and ladder sang out toward the hospital. The boy awakened to see the firefighters climbing through his hospital window. In the arms of one of them, he *asked weakly, "Does this really mean I'm a fireman?" The firefighter responded, "You always were." That night the boy died.*[7]

What can a parent do when a child is born who doesn't match their expectations? It's terribly hard, even scary, to let go of all of the hopes and dreams that have accumulated during pregnancy. Harder still are the moments of uncomfortable silence from friends and family. But staying connected with love is the best safeguard against the fear and hopelessness that can steal our spirit. We can reinvent, reinforce, and express our dreams and love for our children and for each other through ritual and ceremony. Within the special "bubble" of ceremony, we can retool our beliefs and hopes and mobilize our community to support us.

Trusting and loving unconditionally—it's the task of our beginning, and ultimately will be the task of our ending.

SPRING
Adolescence (Ages 14–21)

House made of noon sun
House of strength
Happily may I walk
Happily with abundant showers may I walk
Happily with abundant plants may I walk
Happily on the trail of pollen may I walk
Happily may I walk
—from the Navajo Nightway Chant

T HE TASK OF adolescence is to become independent and find a personal identity. Until this age, you've been your parents' child. Adolescence is the time to learn who else you are. Are you going to be able to "paddle your own canoe"? Do you have the capacity to make decisions and carry them out? Who are you, and what are you made of?

The great American psychologist Erik Erikson described the teenager's work as detaching from the family and constructing a personal identity. The major task at this time is to become his or her own person. This task can be demanding, needing a lot of creative effort from the teenager. Parents who are struggling with their own uncertainties and unfinished business often have trouble helping their kids through this transition.

Some cultures recognize that teens need a moratorium, a period of months, even years, when they can delay their responsibilities and obligations before assuming adult commitments. During this time of transition, teens can actively seek out their identity and attain an understanding of themselves and their culture. This transition is harder in our modern, fast-paced culture, as adolescents move more directly from childhood toward adult concerns and expectations.[1,2] Without clear coming-of-age ceremonies during adolescence, young people can't develop a personal mastery that comes from trying life out. Ceremonies that address these transitions between the seasons of our lives create the setting to focus on new mastery.

The most elaborate of the surviving Apache ceremonies is the female coming of age, "na ih es," which means "getting her ready." The White Painted Woman, the bringer of life, instructs the participants in this annual summer ceremony celebrating a girl's puberty. The young initiate identifies with the White Painted Woman and becomes empowered with her spirit. On the first day, a tipi is constructed; the girl lives there during the four-day ceremony. This structure becomes the center of creation; from here springs forth life, womanhood.

So strong is the initiate's generative power at this time that she is seen as possessing curative qualities. The sick come to her. She touches their bodies, attends to them, prays for them.

During this time the initiate does not smile and laugh, not only because it causes premature wrinkling, but also because it keeps her from thinking powerful thoughts. The survival of her people depends on this ceremony. She is attended by her sponsor, a woman of outstanding qualities whom she will emulate. The maiden initiate carries a sacred wand. This is the staff of life prepared and blessed by Apache holy men. The staff will always remind her of her power, her blessings, her people.

At night the Mountain Spirits visit the maiden, reminding her that she is protected and blessed. At the end of four days, she plants the staff firmly in the ground, as now she is planted in the soil of her culture, and says:

I come to White Painted Woman

By means of long life I come to her

I come to her by means of blessing

I come to her by means of good fortune

I come to her by means of all her different fruits

By means of the long life she bestows, I come to her

By means of this holy path she goes about

White Painted Woman's power emerges

White Painted Woman carries me

She carries me through long life

She carries me to good fortune

She carries me to old age

She bears me to peaceful sleep.[3]

With the abandonment of a nomadic, hunter-warrior lifestyle, the coming-of-age ritual for Apache males is not often performed anymore. The void created by the loss of this and other warrior ceremonies seems to have been filled by extensive alcoholism and violence.

In the coming-of-age ritual, the boy's father would send

him on a quest for vision. The young man would spend a time alone to seek strength, to find a purpose. He would go for days without food or water and armed only with a knife. His father would send him away, as Geronimo's father did, saying:

> You must do something, you run to that mountain and come back, that will make you strong, my son. You know no one is your friend, not even your sister, your father, or your mother. Your legs are your friends, your brain is your friend, your eyesight is your friend, your hair is your friend, your hands are your friends, you must do something with them. Someday you will be with people who are starving, you will have to get something to eat for them. If you go somewhere you must beat the enemy who are attacking you before they get over the hill. Before they beat you, you must get in front of them and bring them back dead. Then all the people will be proud of you, then you will be the only man, then all people will talk about you. That is why I talk to you in this way.[4]

Adolescence has always been a period of permissive tolerance, a time for trying out new behaviors, a time for testing limits while at the same time incorporating the values of the society.[5] The purpose of ceremonies marking adolescence is to instill in the adolescent a feeling of competence, a sense of validation and acceptance. When these ceremonies are lacking, a void is created—a void that must be filled by something. All too often, this void is filled with a jumble of confused values and aspirations that is not life-supporting and ultimately not sustaining. As we strip our culture of ceremonies, myths, and values, we shouldn't be surprised that children's and adolescents' play imitates the adult activities they see around them or the popular "heroes" of their culture. Today, teens' "recreation" seems to be drive-by shootings and other warfare. What does that say about the world they see modeled through television and movies that glorify violence? Adolescent posturing and experimentation have become much more deadly.

Our value system is so poorly defined that we no longer have a clear definition of what is acting out and what is criminal. Without guidance and rituals to introduce the challenges of adulthood, adolescents are acting out their fantasies indiscriminately, which is why suicide and homicide account for one-third of all deaths in this age group.[6,7,8]

In 1990, among 15-to-24-year-olds, 12,607 deaths occurred from motor vehicle accidents, 7,354 deaths from homicide, and 4,869 deaths from suicide—accounting for 68 percent of all deaths in this age group. Of the suicides, 85 percent were males. Suicide rates in the 15-to-19-year-old group more than doubled from 1970 to 1990.[9]

Cultures with intact initiation rituals that promote the work of adolescence do not have high death rates from crime, suicide, or homicide. These rituals provide a safe and positive context in which to "act out" and, in so doing, to move through adolescence into adulthood. Cultures that devalue ceremonies promoting time-honored values and beliefs leave their people more vulnerable during the hard times. Even if the rituals are basic—for example, shared mealtimes and holiday observances—they serve as a powerful force to promote unity and connectedness and, paradoxically, individuality. In families with few or no ritual observances, there is a much greater occurrence of alcoholism than in families in which even these simple rituals were continued.[10]

Without guidance, adolescents create their own rituals and values with their own dress, symbols, language, beliefs, and blessings. Because they are created by the adolescents themselves, they do not contain good advice, values, or perspective about the future. Without clear values, it's hard to get through this stage of life. One of Howard's colleagues who works with teenagers in trouble told the following story:

On the day of his initiation, Danny felt a mixture of pride and fear. Today would be the day he would become a man. He adjusted his cap to be sure it looked just right and slipped out of the house. As he walked down the street, he nervously fumbled with the 9mm semiautomatic pistol in his pocket. Sure, he had fired it many times before, but he had never shot it at another person.

He wound through the neighborhood and went inside an abandoned apartment house where the gang initiation would take place. As he entered the building, he felt another pang of excitement and dread. Inside, the members of the gang were gathering. "You ready?" asked the leader of the group. "Yeah, sure," Danny replied. In a corner of the room, several other members were smoking crack in a well-used glass pipe. "Take a few hits and get fired up—today's a special day, you know!" said one of the group. As the smoke filled his lungs, Danny felt a rush of exhilaration. This was his group, his tribe, and soon he would become a full member.

The leader announced that it was time to begin their initiation. He dipped his index finger in the ashes in the bowl of the pipe and traced a small circle on the forehead of each of the initiates and declared, "We ain't nothin' alone, but together we have the power to stop the world. Do you accept this power?" Each of them said, "Yes!" Then he extinguished a lit cigarette inside the circle of ashes on their foreheads.

They loaded everybody into the back seat of an old Chevrolet the leader drove. At first they wound through their neighborhood slowly, displaying their colors until they were sufficiently pumped to enter their rivals' territory.

The car picked up speed as they raced past a corner where a bunch of young men were hanging out. Danny leaned out and began firing his pistol until he ran out of bullets. Only then did he realize he had closed his eyes before shooting. Everybody was yelling and screaming with excitement as they returned to their lair.

The initiation ceremony changed Danny. Somehow from that time on, Danny was fearless. Even though he was only five feet tall, nobody dared to mess with him. He carried his pistol as a badge of courage and displayed it as a sign of one who had been initiated. But it didn't take long for Danny to have trouble with the law. Eventually, he was referred to a rehabilitation program. After a few months in various groups, Danny was ready for the ropes course.

The ropes course is created as a symbol for a young person's life. Those who go through the course climb upward past their fears and limits, connected by ropes to the peers who support them physically and emotionally. The course models commitment, responsibility, support, and possibility. The participants learn how to express their points of view without making other people wrong. The physical challenges force them to find the balance between being independent and being able to follow rules and instructions. They can transform their past and symbolically create a vision for the future.

The course starts with a "warmup" consisting of ground-level events. These games and events are designed to build trust, communication, and support. The kids get used to being touched in safe and supportive ways. They lift each other and spot for each other. Even the roughest, toughest guys begin to give each other hugs.

None of the events is only about climbing to the top. Achieving the top of the ropes course is about going one step further than you think you can go. It is about confronting fear, but it's more than that. It's choosing whether to go or stop based on your own decision as opposed to responding to fear or your peers calling the shots.

Danny came to the event called the pole. The pole is thirty feet straight up and is climbed on staples. On the top is a platter that's about ten inches in diameter. To get down from the top, you jump in the air to catch a trapeze.

Danny's friends helped him put on his helmet and checked his harness to be sure it was on properly. They attached the safety ropes to his harness and gave the other ends to the belayers who would support him if he fell. He stood at the base of the pole and saluted his belayers. He then announced to the group, "I choose to climb this pole . . . belayers ready?" They replied crisply, "Yes!" Danny then announced, "Danny is climbing," as he carefully worked his way up the pole one step at a time.

Danny got about five staples up, about ten feet off the ground, and completely fell apart. It was not because of his fear of heights; he realized that he was doing something he didn't think he could do, and it was conflicting with the way he had made other decisions in his life. He had always said, "This is the way it is because . . ." but he wasn't able to make those kinds of rationalizations when he was climbing the pole. When he got to seven staples, he said he had done the best he could. But by accepting the support and coaching of the group and by focusing in on his commitment to go as far as he could, *he managed to climb to the top of the pole. He took a deep breath, jumped, and caught the trapeze. When he hit the ground, he was a different kid. He knew that he was more than his gang identity. He could accept support from others; he could be depended upon by others; he believed that if it was believed possible to complete these events, it was possible to do whatever he committed himself to.*

Two and a half years later, he's going to school and has his own apartment.

Gang involvement provides adolescents with community, ceremony, and ritual; however, all too often the values that are promoted are negative and the ceremonies ultimately are self-destructive.

Another modern self-destructive ritual is the eating disorder. The premium on appearance is so intense that teens torture themselves into binge eating and then vomiting, or they undergo long periods of self-induced starvation. Some young women alternate between the two.[11] These self-destructive behaviors are symptoms of the pressures derived from a culture whose definitions of worth and power are based on material superficiality. These shallow values fail to provide teenagers with guidance for establishing a stable identity.

How can we help create healing rituals for this season, for kids starved for values and guidance? Howard was witness to the following dramatic event:

Rabbi Bill Berk went to see a 14-year-old girl who had been admitted to the hospital in the late phase of anorexia weighing less than 90 pounds. She had been in and out of a multitude of treatment programs with little benefit. Her parents, in desperation, had phoned the rabbi to see if he would talk with Terry in the hospital. Perhaps he could reach her in some way.

In a moment of inspiration, he brought with him a Torah, the most sacred totemic object in the Jewish faith. He placed it on a chair in the corner of Terry's room and they talked. She promised to do better, to try eating more, etc., etc.

The rabbi sensed that her endless repetition of these promises wasn't sincere. Suddenly and without warning, he held her and began to weep. He did not know why he was so overcome by sadness at the moment, and this behavior surprised them both. Apparently, nobody had ever expressed concern for her in such a way before. Rabbi Berk picked up the Torah and handed it to Terry. She cradled it in her arms and started to cry, saying she often prayed to God to keep her small. "God does not want us to be small," the rabbi responded. "He wants us to grow. Growing means not just seeing yourself as your imperfections. Stand tall when you pray because you are so beautiful." And they both cried until Terry looked up and said, "I want to eat lunch," and they both laughed. When lunch came, they recited the blessing before meals, she holding the Torah in one arm and her fork in the other, shoveling away. "It tastes good," she said. "You know, I haven't tasted anything in years until I tasted the salt in your tears. Then I knew God loved me anyway."

Terry left the hospital, went back to school, and has done well ever since.

You don't have to be in trouble in order to ceremonialize your life. Sometimes the most powerful ceremonies can be the simplest, as Howard relates:

From the beginning, Sharona and I had a custom that we would sit down together for dinner. When we had kids, we sat down as a family. It wasn't always easy, sometimes not even pleasant, but dinnertime was always a special event. We said a blessing before we ate as a reminder about what we were thankful for. It could be something that touched your heart, something you saw or learned. Dinnertime evolved into the focal point of our family life. Everyone spoke about the highlights of their day.

From our "dinner table highlights," we developed something we called "family meetings." If things got heavy and problematic issues demanded more than dinnertime highlights, anybody could call a family meeting. We had two simple rules. First, when one person talked, everybody else listened until that person was finished. Second, discussion did not end until the person who asked for the family meeting felt that he or she had reached some closure.

Last summer we were planning a family vacation to Colorado. Our younger teenage daughter decided to make an audio tape of her favorite songs to play in the car on the long drive there. Soon we began to hear voices being raised in our family room, and before very long we could hear her arguing loudly with her older sister. "I don't like the songs on your tape!" shouted our older daughter. By the time we broke up the fight, they were both in tears. We'll discuss this tonight at dinner at a family meeting—until then, you will both need to think about how to work this out! we told them.

That night at dinner, both teenage daughters presented their points of view and, as is our custom, we all listened. Then we decided as a group that each daughter would make a list of the songs she liked and they would make two tapes together containing all of their choices. They also decided that each of them would record her sister's selections. It became pretty obvious that they would have to work together and *find a way to compromise on their musical choices. The final tapes were a wonderful treat to listen to all the way to Colorado and back!*

These family ceremonies bonded us together. They taught us all how to confront differences in an atmosphere that promotes a willingness to listen and how to always reconnect with each other.

A ceremony can capture the potential of a moment and propel us forward. Whether it's Danny's leap from the climbing pole, Terry's leap of faith, or the family members communicating with each other in mutual love and respect, the adolescent is able to separate from being a child while remaining connected to the tribe and to the tree of life. Through sharing this experience, others can feel a sense of awe and see expanded possibilities for themselves.

EARLY SUMMER
Early Adulthood (Ages 22–35)

House made of noon sun

Happily may I walk

with abundant showers

with abundant plants

on a trail of pollen

Happily may I walk

—from the Navajo

Nightway Chant

EARLY ADULTHOOD IS the time of plenty, of excitement that comes with new possibilities, believable dreams, independence, making our own choices, and creating our own opportunities.[1,2] It can also be a time of trouble, because what we've learned so far may not have prepared us well to undertake the continued journey of life. We may have accumulated such heavy burdens in childhood and adolescence that those old teachings won't leave, and they limit our ability to enjoy the choices and the abundance of adulthood.

Some of us have been taught to believe that we will "never amount to anything" or are "born to lose." Sometimes we learn the opposite: "There's nothing you can't do" or

"You'll always be the best." Sooner or later, whatever the messages we received while growing up, most of us discover that we are flawed and imperfect. While the support (or lack of support) we received influences how we cope with the realization, sometimes we're not great (which doesn't mean we're bad). Coming to peace with this assault on our egos is the work of adulthood.

Storytelling—a ritual that involves sharing of experience—is the oldest healing art. Telling and listening to each other's stories is how we make sense of our own life experiences. As soon as we say "once upon a time," "imagine," or "remember when," we set the stage to focus our attention on new possibilities and ways of learning. There is a healing, nurturing relationship between storyteller and listener. A ceremony can be a vehicle for telling a new story, or retelling an old one, and often telling a story is a ceremony in itself.

The reason Bible stories, folk tales, and fairy tales are so powerful and appealing is that they tell tales every human being can relate to, generation after generation.[3] Storytellers enter into a passionate trance that induces listeners to pay attention. By weaving a mesmerizing, spellbinding tale, storytellers hook our imagination, and using the imagination makes dreams possible.

Engaging with each other through listening to each other's stories is how we refocus on our lives, get new ideas, and feel new hope. Stories help us consider that there may be other ways of doing, feeling, thinking, and behaving. By listening to a story, we can take a step away from our current lives.

The first step a healer must take in helping us create

change is to get our attention. It may take a long time to get you to pay attention. Old learning is so ingrained and new possibilities so dim that, without realizing it, we may be colluding in giving up our dreams before giving them a shot.

Milton Erickson, a legendary psychiatrist and hypno-therapist, discovered that he could get his patients' attention by telling a seemingly unrelated story or some delightful bit of humor. They'd wonder what he was trying to tell them, and that wonder would begin the process of opening their minds to new possibilities. His stories often sent his listeners on a search into their unconscious minds to discover some new way of understanding what he was saying.[4,5,6]

This process—looking again at something we thought we knew—is what gives rise to every creative breakthrough. Every act of genius or insight is simply the result of a pre-pared mind and a serendipitous event.

In a flash we can become enlightened, if we are prepared to harvest the miraculous moment.

A storyteller can open us up to that creative moment, when old unconscious associations get suspended and new light can fill our lives. Stories can help to heal our minds as well. Psychotherapy is a storytelling ceremony through which people see their light.

Among the Hawaiian natives, storytellers are called "Maolis," which means "Light Carriers." They tell tales about creation, about how and why things are the way they are. The Maolis say:

Each child at birth is given a bowl of perfect light. If you tend your light, it will grow in strength and you can do all things (swim with sharks, fly with birds, know and understand all things). If, however, you become envious or jealous, you drop a stone into your bowl of light and some of the light goes out. If you become violent, another stone is dropped in; cruel, another stone; and so on and on. Light and a stone cannot occupy the same space. If you continue to put stones in your bowl of light, the light will go out and then you will become a stone.[7]

Stones can neither grow nor move by themselves. But human beings can at any time, if they tire of being stones, choose to turn their bowls upside down, and the stones will fall away and the light will grow again.

The work of adulthood is rediscovering the light within us. We all carry stones: stones of doubt, fear, and other old learnings that anchor us in the past. We can, if we choose, relieve ourselves of those burdens. That's what psychotherapy does—help us get rid of the stones picked up since childhood. It's also what twelve-step programs, meditation, journaling, art, and other similar experiences do—help us to grow.

You probably already have the answers you seek; you just don't see them. Psychotherapy sets the stage so you can pay attention and uncover what you already know, but don't know that you know. You change behavior by letting go of the old and moving on. Growth has nothing to do with adding on; it has to do with letting go.

Human beings are the only species that can choose *not* to let go. We may know our behavior is dysfunctional (like having a short temper, being alcoholic, or seeking out people who hurt us), but we often keep doing the same old things in the same old way because we don't believe we can do it differently. Animals can't hang on to their dysfunctions. When it's time for deer to shed their antlers, they don't say, "I've grown accustomed to these antlers. Oh, I know they're not great, one side has a branch missing and the others are blunted; but it's what I've got and it would just be my luck that if I shed these I'd get some fungal infection and then no new ones would grow back at all. I want to be attractive! Something is better than nothing, and I can't have everything."

There are always reasons to hang on to the old behaviors and beliefs, even if they don't work anymore. But in adulthood, we must let go of the old dysfunctional behaviors in order to grow. When we let go, we're left vulnerable for a while. If we're unwilling to be vulnerable and to take risks, we'll never grow. Vulnerability is simply an opportunity for new learning.

As storytellers, psychiatrists help to weave a tapestry that can show us our lives in a new way, without fear, strengthening us in our vulnerability. Sadly, like other medical specialists, psychiatrists today spend less time listening and talking with people. We're pressured to work quickly and get immediate results. We spend less time with our patients and prescribe more drugs.[8]

Medication isn't always the answer. The best way to get rid of old accumulated stories and make the journey into adulthood is by creating dreams based on today's truth, not yesterday's promises. We need to empty the bowl so we can see new light; otherwise we will be immobilized. Carl's patient, Peter, had some "old stories" to rewrite:

Peter was an affluent, upper-middle-class, brilliant physicist who was married with children. Though he seemed to have everything and was a success by outward standards, he suffered from an obsessive-compulsive disorder. He not only worried about how much money he had or how much his wife was spending—he called the bank daily, obsessed about lost deposit slips; he couldn't go to bed unless he reconciled his bank balance to the penny.

At night he would stay awake wondering if he had closed the refrigerator door tightly enough. Sooner or later he would go downstairs to check it. He knew he had shut the door, but he couldn't help himself.

In college, Peter experienced obsessions and compulsions also. He sat in the front row of every class. He became famous on campus for his scrupulous notes, which other students would copy and study, acing their final exams even if they'd never gone to class. He couldn't deny students access to his notes because he couldn't bear not to please them.

By the time he went to college, Peter "knew" that sooner or later he would fail and some disaster would befall him. He prepared himself for this inevitable eventuality by creating little rituals to alleviate his anxiety. He would start the day reciting magical names that had to begin with the first letter of the first word in the title of the first song he heard when he was awakened by his clock radio. Then he had to step on the "right" bathroom tiles, or something bad would happen that day. He believed that if he ever got the rituals down right, he could ultimately control every outcome in his life.

Even though he knew in his conscious mind that things happened over which he had no control, this had no impact on his behavior. When Peter came to me for help, it took a year before he trusted me enough to say something he felt rather than something he thought would please me. He wanted to be the perfect patient. Slowly he ventured to try new ways.

One night he went to a movie with some close friends. He hated the film, so in the middle of the movie he left but didn't tell anyone he was leaving. In the lobby, he anguished about his decision. Perhaps he should have told somebody. They'll worry, they'll be mad. Was there something in the movie that he didn't see or appreciate?

When the movie was over, his wife and friends emerged and asked him why he'd left. Over coffee, he told them that the subject of the movie—the seduction of a young girl by a middle-aged business-man—frankly disgusted him. The friends wondered if his reaction had something to do with his feelings about his adolescent daughter. Maybe, he said, but that didn't make him like the movie any more. "Okay," his friends said. "You didn't like it."

That was it, and the subject was dropped. It was over, without recriminations or judgment. Peter didn't feel rejected or humiliated; his opinion was his, and it was at least as important as theirs. That single spontaneous act of passion, which took two years of psycho-therapy to achieve, marked the beginning of Peter's ability to reexamine his old beliefs.

In adulthood, we learn to recognize and accept our lim-itations and recognize the things we can't control. Only then can we pursue our possibilities. Psychotherapy itself can be a safe and secure ceremony through which we can identify and make new choices, allowing us to begin creating a healthier and more satisfying life story.

Psychotherapy is a ceremony in which we talk about our fears, hopes, and innermost secrets. With guidance, it helps us rekindle our spirits. There are many ways to get help to look at our old certainties in new ways.

Every summer, the tribes of the Great Plains hold their sacred Sundance whose central theme is the renewal of the world. When a man makes a vow to Sundance, he pledges not only for himself but also his family and tribe to ensure their place in the universe.

The Sundance takes eight days. The first four are spent alone, during which one prays and reflects on how to walk on the earth in a good way, how to walk in beauty, how to fulfill the promise to the Creator for having given him a tribe.

The last four days are devoted to the building of the altar, to dancing and self-sacrifice. Sacrificial flesh offerings are made by the pledgers in pursuit of enlightenment. They pierce through the skin of their chests with wooden pegs and then suspend themselves from the Sacred Tree, which is their altar. The pledgers make this flesh offering as the only thing they have to give that truly belongs to them. Through making this sacrifice, their spirit becomes one with the Great Spirit, who can grant peace and harmony to the planet. They pray for a time when all on the earth shall come together as relatives.

No one dies from this or even suffers long after. Their tribe members look at the pledgers with respect for the sincere way they give thanks to Wakan Tanka, The Great Spirit, for sustaining life and abundance.

In the beginning of the twentieth century, the government outlawed the Sundance as a barbaric ritual. The offering of living flesh as a sacrifice was deemed "a degenerate and primitive practice" apparently. But the tribes continued the ceremony anyway. Eventually they petitioned the courts, saying that they needed to fulfill this sacred obligation if they were to survive. It was only with the passage of the Native American Religious Freedoms Act in 1978 that public piercing was again legal and didn't have to be practiced secretly.

The Sundance takes place in a "sacred hoop," a circle about fifty yards in diameter, at the center of which stands a tree that is perhaps fifty feet tall. Each Sundancer attaches his own rope to the tree. It is from this rope, his spiritual lifeline to the Great Spirit, that he will suspend himself during the ordeal.

Only the men pierce themselves; it is taught that women give their blood every month to sustain life on the planet, and men only give blood at this time. Once a dancer has tied his rope, it must be used; otherwise his spirit cannot be released. If a dancer becomes sick and cannot pierce, then someone else must pierce for him, to release his soul.

When it is a dancer's turn to pierce, he is brought to the base of the pole. After he lies down on a buffalo hide, parallel incisions are made on both sides of his chest or back (sometimes both) and a thumb-width strip of skin is lifted. Under this a sharpened spike is thrust; the dancers do not cry out. The dancer's rope is fastened to these pegs. Then the dancer stands up and walks slowly backwards until the rope is taut. Leaning backwards, he dances until his skin tears loose. That moment of release, every dancer says, is one of liberation.

Today, there are places where non-Indians have participated in the Sundance. These are people who are familiar with the culture, and whose commitment and spirit have been deemed worthy. Carl knows such a man:

I call him my "son." He has been a mental health consultant among the Great Plains tribes for more than twenty years; his specialty is in addictionology. He works with hard-core addicts and criminals (pedophiles, rapists, and wife beaters). His commitment to bearing human suffering is enormous.

His wife left him because she didn't want to compete for his attention with every other needy cause. He rationalized her leaving by telling himself that he didn't deserve her anyway. I asked him whether it didn't have more to do with his inability to ever allow himself to feel good. It didn't matter how often we'd talk or I'd beat him over the head with my insight; he never gave up clients who had learned to depend on him. He could find a way to be suckled on demand. He identified with hopeless causes even at the expense of his health.

Eventually he became depressed. He sought out his Spiritual Father, a Lakota medicine man, who told him he needed to spend four days "in the ground." That meant he was to be buried alive in a hole into which a hollow pipe was thrust so that he could breathe. It was a ceremony few, except Shamans, endured and I told him he was crazy. You don't have to suffer more, I said, you have to live more. But he decided to prepare himself for a year before undertaking this purification ordeal.

When they dug him out, he told me he finally understood what it meant to be alone. From that moment on, he vowed to reach out and ask for more for himself. He took more time off from work. He fell in love and remarried.

As part of his marital vows, he pledged to his Spiritual Father that he wanted to Sundance and to thank God for his liberation.

For the following year he tied a thousand "tobacco ties," which are sacred prayer bundles. He went to weekly sweat lodge ceremonies and learned to sing the Sundance songs. During this time he also gathered the elements required for participation.

I sent him an eagle feather that had been given to me by a rabbi friend who used it as the "pointer" while reading the Torah. I told my son about the significance of this feather that had moved between the lines of Torah and therefore carried the prayers of my tribe to touch the ear of God.

It was that feather that he tied to the rope that suspended him from the Sacred Tree. Feathers that are tied to the piercing ropes are later given away. Anyone who is seeking some kind of healing can enter the dance grounds and participate. This ceremony-within-the-ceremony takes place on the third day of Sundance.

To receive such a feather is highly prized because each one is filled with the spirit of a true believer.

It was the feather that he focused on during his piercing. It hung down from his rope right into the middle of his view of the afternoon sun. In the wind he saw it dancing, and in his pain he remembered something I'd once told him about his never being able to experience enough pain. In that moment he understood that the only way to get beyond his pain was to be truly with it now in its enormity and then break through it.

He later wrote:

I have finally freed myself from pain. I was looking at that rabbi's feather you gave me, it was dancing in the sun and I heard that stuff you used to lay on me about no pain too great and that I could give it up. When I saw the feather dance with pain it became clear to me that I wanted to dance with joy and then I knew I had finally gotten beyond it.

~

61

As I read, I thought, insight can prepare the mind for change, but ceremony can unleash its power.

He gave that feather away to one of his patients. She was a chronically abused woman with whom he had worked for years. He blessed her with it, waving smoke from burning cedar all over her. He handed it to her and then said that to break away from that tree he realized it was only himself who could do it. He told her he had helped her all he could, and now she had to break her chains. This feather would help her, he said.

Ceremonial acts are more effective than words because they help us get another perspective on ourselves. They can even provide us with strategies for handling suffering.

Ceremonies can create a safe place to make new choices. They can release guilt and shame. The Catholic ceremony of confession is a wonderful example of a powerful method of doing this. Some find more creative ways: This story appeared in *The Minneapolis Star Tribune*:

Five women gathered in the chapel of the Roman Catholic Church of St. Therese in Deephaven. Each of them had an abortion. Now they gathered with a Catholic deacon.

Each woman named her aborted child and then commended its soul to someone in heaven. One woman chose Mary, because the mother of Jesus had given up her son too. Others chose a grandparent long since departed. They read scripture, cried, and eventually turned over their pain to a God they prayed would forgive them.

There are many sacred places of healing and refuge where one can face one's truth and be able to move on.

When the choices we have made no longer are viable for us, we must move on and let go of the old. The following story about letting go also appeared in *The Minneapolis Star Tribune*:

A couple stood at a church altar to ceremonialize their divorce. The minister asked each of them, "In the presence of God, do you now relinquish your status as husband and wife, thus freeing you from all responsibilities to each other except those that you willingly give to another child of God?"

Each one answered in turn, "I do."

Their marriage had ended formally a month earlier, but it didn't seem quite finished. So they gathered with friends and relatives and observed the end of their twenty-one-year marriage in the church.

With tears in their eyes, their friends spoke to them, one at a time, saying how glad they were that these two had chosen to share their pain and their forgiveness so openly. Then the minister welcomed them both back to the United Methodist Church.

Sometimes, young adulthood is the end of the journey. Then we must face the shadow of death prematurely, as David Kalish's Associated Press story from November 12, 1995, reveals:

It was drizzling in Brooklyn's Prospect Park, and I ran as if chased. My shadow jumped across the lamplighted road, jerking from tree to tree. I veered around puddles. Drops splattered my face. Sooner than usual, the brownstones of Park Slope reassured me that I had arrived home.

It had been only an imagined Grim Reaper spooking me to run faster. But relief mingled with my sweat as I slowed to a walk. My legs had outraced the sort of fear that few people conjure on routine runs. Imagining the worst was more than a handy motivator. It affirmed why I was training for this year's New York City Marathon.

Two Aprils ago, I was diagnosed with a rare, incurable form of thyroid cancer. A finisher of five marathons in the 1980s, I was stunned that years of fitness had proven so little protection against disease. Through two operations and accompanying emotional trauma, however, hope gradually built that a grueling running regimen might help me surmount more than just the 26-mile course.

My decision followed a series of extraordinary events. I remember sitting in a doctor's office, tears rolling down my cheeks from the pain of a tube stuck down my nose. The image from a tiny camera at the end made the doctor sigh heavily, then tell me the lump in my throat was "no doubt" malignant. One week earlier I'd lost half my voice, permanently I learned later when doctors explained that the tumor on my thyroid had wrapped around my left laryngeal vocal nerve. My fit self-image was further eroded by operations, the most recent in April. All told, I lost my thyroid, lymph nodes and various structures from both sides of my neck.

Still, the surgeon couldn't get everything. Blood tests indicate that imperceptible cancer cells persist in my body, and since the cancer had reached my lymph nodes, chances are rogue cells have traveled outside my neck and I live with the threat of recurrence. Medullary thyroid cancer generally does not respond to chemotherapy and radiation, the primary treatment is further surgery. For now, my disease is inactive, and I feel healthy.

Shortly after the April surgery, as I recuperated at my father's beachfront apartment on Long Island, more marathon seeds sprouted. On the fourth day out of the hospital I tried a short jog. I was *amazed how invigorated I felt so soon after surgery. I told a friend I wanted to conquer something that seemed insurmountable. Marathon training, I figured, would somehow steel me against the chance the lingering cancer inside me would act up again before a cure can be found.*

The reality of training was more perspiration than glory. If I was somehow reclaiming my immortality, I was not aware of it trudging halfway across Brooklyn, sweat freeze-drying on my neck at an hour when most people are wrestling bedsheets. But sometimes I felt more deeply satisfied than during my 1980s training. Sometimes passing scenery appears sharper and lingers longer, as if I am observing for the first time. I notice this one morning approaching the Brighton Beach boardwalk. The Atlantic Ocean looks solid and blue. Sand whips across the boardwalk slats, seeming to smolder in the sun. I pass an abandoned Coney Island roller coaster. On a concrete wall, sculpted fish smile strangely. I run across the nearly deserted beach. Perhaps, I later think, I feel a sadness for what I may not someday see again.

In April, just before my second operation, I traveled 3,000 miles to try to leave behind such anxieties. I went alone to Mexico for a week, to a new Pacific Coast resort. Gardeners stared from under broad hats as I jogged by sunburnt jungle. I was still sweating when I returned to my hotel room. I slid open the balcony doors. The crash of ocean was everywhere, its symphony soaring over palm trees and strolling couples.

I recalled that sound two weeks later as I lay in my hospital bed, afraid to move my head. It was 4:30 a.m., half a day after my surgeon had removed about 50 lymph nodes from my neck.

Tonight, I run alone through Prospect Park. The race is days away. Yellowed leaves reflect across the lake's dark surface, and I wonder if I am prepared. There are many things to think about. I feel that things are settling down. I've finally refurnished my apartment. After the race I am returning to Mexico to try out months of Spanish lessons. Dry leaves rattle behind me, just to my left. It's probably a squirrel eager for acorns. But I imagine my hooded pursuer testing my flank, black shoes sneaking up. Anything is possible at this point, but I hold out for the final stretch.

The work of early adulthood is making, repairing, and communicating choices that define yourself now. So what do sundancing and marathon training have in common? They are the ceremonial events through which the hero's call to action is acted out. It celebrates a willingness to cross the threshold into uncertainty and fear and emerge victorious and transformed.

You don't have to be Odysseus shipwrecked on the Island of One-Eyed Giants, Beowulf slaying Grendel, or Braveheart staked out before his enemies. We all get a chance to face the fear monsters of our lives. We face them with added courage and dignity if we tread the ceremonial path that helps us find the strength to undertake the hero's journey.

LATE SUMMER
Maturity (Ages 36–55)

House made of darkening clouds
Dark Cloud is at House's door
The trail out of it is darkened
The zigzag lightning stands high upon it
Happily may I walk
with abundant showers
with abundant plants
on a trail of pollen
Happily may I walk
—from the Navajo Nightway Chant

BY AGE 35, we've all had some successes and some fail-
ures. If we haven't stumbled by now, we haven't walked
very far. By the time we reach our mature years, we've probably tried things that didn't work out, experienced things that
left us humbled, and confronted pain.

The task of maturity is to acquire a sense of proportion,
a realistic appraisal of who we are and our relationship with
the rest of the world.[1] It is to stop measuring ourselves by a
previous standard of what we thought we had to be or
achieve to feel successful. This means letting go of some of

our earlier standards for success or completeness. Maturity is the time to reconcile earlier dreams with today's reality. The way we hoped it would be is not necessarily the way it is or will be. Carl knew a high school hero who lettered in three sports:

He was popular, good-looking, and smart, and I envied him. At a reunion, I saw him again. He was pot-bellied, working a job in town, and drinking too much. I learned he had never finished college or become the professional baseball player he aimed to be. Years later, he still believed the most productive time of his life ended when he graduated from high school.

The loss of a parent may force us toward this reconciliation quickly, as Howard and his cousin discovered together:

After my father died, the family gathered at my mom's home to "sit shiva." This ancient Jewish mourning ritual includes friends and family gathering for seven days to help family through the most intense period of transition and mourning following a loss.

I was sitting at the kitchen table with several close family members. Other people drifted in and out as we wove stories about the old days, my father and other relatives who had passed. I started talking with my eldest cousin, Rick. He had just turned fifty the year before, and we had given him an AARP membership at a surprise party thrown by his wife. Pretty soon, we began talking about his father. Several years ago, he had been visiting his dad. They were outside showing one of his father's classic cars to a potential buyer when his father suddenly dropped to the ground, dying instantly from a massive heart attack. Rick had attempted to resuscitate him, but by the time the paramedics arrived, it was too late. Rick was always a joker, but we shared our stories and our grief at this special time in a special and serious way. He confessed, "I am the oldest cousin. My children come to me for advice—me, can you believe it? What do I tell them? Do I have the experience to be the elder in the family?" I nodded and said, "Yes, it is a frightening thing, becoming the family elder. But what choice do we have? Time goes on, and we grow into new roles. Let's hope our fathers have prepared us well!" Rick nodded and we sat silently together, watching our kids as they talked and laughed together at the table next to us.

If we only hang on to old certainties, we'll never know if new dreams can come true. The past is a building block to the future, but we have to leave the past behind in order to grow and change. The work of maturity is to silence the ego long enough to have a word with ourselves and reexamine everything we once thought we knew. It is especially important to look at how we perceive ourselves and our place in the world.

Ours is a culture that lauds youth and has no formal ceremony for honoring the process of becoming an elder. In such a culture, it becomes easy to wallow in self-pity as we age. This season cannot be denied by plastic surgery, muscular development, running marathons, or seducing hard bodies—it can only be delayed. The task of late summer is to learn to love ourselves for what we are, not for what we believe we ought to be. Part of choosing who we want to be involves beginning to prepare ourselves for the eventual transformation into an elder. Like the adolescent, the mature adult must let go of the old story and make the transition into the new one. One way of marking this transition into elder status is to craft a special ceremony, as Howard recounts:

The elders in our congregation had studied the wisdom literature of our faith for nearly four years. Over the course of the final two years, they met weekly to write about their life experiences and spiritual selves. At the end of this intense time of study, reflection and sharing, they truly had earned the title of "elder."

To mark this transition, we held a special service of dedication for them. The room was crowded with family and friends. A special canopy was held by the elders as five- and six-year-old children were consecrated into the congregation. Then the elders were placed under the canopy and special prayers were said. Their own journal entries were read, marking their transition into wisdom and elder status.

In Indian country, adults acquire a new name in their mature years. Names are chosen to reflect significant changes as the individual goes through life. Among the Hopi, Sioux, Cheyenne, Blackfoot, and many other tribes, people were traditionally called by several names. Each name had special meaning, reflecting some specific experience, talent, or accomplishment.

Choosing a new name as an adult lets you present yourself to the world as the person you now see yourself to be. Why be called by a name that no longer fits? Ceremonies during adulthood allow the community to recognize and reinforce the identity described in the new story.

In the Hopi adult naming ceremony, the person is fully initiated into kachina society. He will sit in the kiva facing the Sipapu in the east, the symbolic hole through which the Hopi first emerged into this world. The kachina chief runs a line of cornmeal from that hole to each initiate. He blesses him with a new name. He tells him, "This line connects you to all of your people, even those who came before. This is now the name by which your ancestors will greet you when you are released from this place to go into the next universe as a kachina."

Carl told this story to a friend of his whom he met at a lecture in Utah's Wasatch Mountains. The change of names has more transformative power when it is done in a public way, as this story depicts:

After the lecture, I hiked to a spectacular mountain pasture with my old friend, Chip, who now calls himself Charles. The summer meadow was a gigantic quilt, a multicolor patchwork of flowers, a celestial hopscotch game on which mountain spirits played.

I'd known him as Chip, so I teased him. "Perhaps I should now call you Sir Charles," I said in a crisp British falsetto accent. He looked at me and said, "All these years that you've known me, there are some things you still don't know." He told me he had recently focused on a life event he thought he had long ago shelved into emotional obscurity.

He knew his birth mother had been a skid row alcoholic who had given him up for adoption just before her death when he was nine. What he didn't want to remember was that she had fondled his genitals. She would talk to them, even kiss them. When he became sick, the first thing she did was to examine his genitals. Her name for him was Chipper; she said it was how he made her feel. His friends called him Chip.

He'd never known his biological father, who had died in World

War II and was named Charles. His adoptive parents had continued to call him Chip. But at age 40, he'd decided to give up this old name because it no longer made him feel good. He'd begun to understand how his lifelong conflicts with women were tied in with his mother's abuse of him, and he wanted to start over in relationships and to be known by a name not associated with his mother.

Throughout his life, Charles had struggled to understand why he was so terrified of intimacy. Twice he'd married women who followed orders. He called the shots, he held control. He didn't understand it was a way to guard against a woman's violence. But once he got control, his wives no longer interested and excited him, and both marriages ended. Now, facing his childhood trauma, he better understood some underpinnings of his conflicts with women.

I told him about the Hopi naming ceremony and Charles immediately asked if he could adapt it. He beamed at the idea. We crafted the ceremony right there in the meadow. He made a list of friends, some of whom lived quite a distance from him. We created an invitation, picked some dates. I agreed to help run the event. We asked people not to bring gifts; instead, their gift would be to come with a name that truly reflected how they saw themselves at this time in their lives.

Eighteen people sat in a circle on Charles's living room floor. In the middle of the circle was a small Indian blanket atop which rested an abalone shell filled with cedar, a burning candle, and a pair of epaulets—the last remnants from his father's military uniform and the only thing of his father's that Charles had. Charles first told the Utah mountain meadow story and how he had shared with me a long-repressed event. He told the story of his childhood and ended by saying he wanted to take his father's name.

Then he said, "These shoulder boards will come to each of you, *and while you're holding them, I'd like you to share the gift you brought me today. Tell me the name you chose for yourself. Nobody will ask why or interpret; each of us will get a turn."*

He handed the epaulets to me, and I said a little about the Talking Circle, about creating a sacred space. I lit the sage, saying it gave color and smell so we could see our words rise to touch the ear of the Creator. I told about my grandson's naming and thought about my father, about great-grandchildren, and about dying. I am Abraham, the son of Aaron. My grandson is Aaron, and one day I hope, someone will carry my name, too. . . .

When I finished, I passed the epaulets on. Some chose names with colors, others with animals. There was one historical figure, and one said she just wanted to be called Mom.

That's how Chip became Charles, his father's son. This is how the power of ceremony can redefine ourselves as adults. By this time of life, experience has taught us that we have, at best, only limited control over our lives. By now, we serve a role in our circle of relatives and friends. But we continue to struggle to sort out which parts of our old stories to keep and which to let go.

Some people, like Chip, use ceremony to move from their past into the present. Others need to harmonize the present with the future. Women at this age often face difficulty in reconciling their physical and emotional cravings to have children with their current life stories.[2] The press of time is felt acutely as women move toward the cessation of their biological childbearing years. In old times, healers would prepare potions and amulets to help couples to conceive. Today, conception can become highly medicalized, virtually removing the woman from the process. By reclaiming her role of creator, Carl's patient Molly was able to achieve her dream and more:

Unless you've been through it, you can't really know how painful it is to face infertility. My struggle for a child brought me face to face with my worst fears about myself. But I would take that journey again in a heartbeat, not just to have my precious son, but to discover what I learned about myself.

At 33, after four years of marriage, I wanted to have a baby. What began as a pretty normal desire became an obsession after a few unsuccessful months. After nearly a year of trying on our own, my husband and I found a fertility doctor who was on the cutting edge of the latest treatments. Although his manner was coldly clinical and a little off-putting, he had "Science" on his side. As long as he could bring me a baby, I didn't care if he wasn't so pleasant to be around.

Within a year, I became pregnant twice, once for two weeks and once for fourteen weeks. Losing the baby at fourteen weeks was the hardest thing I had ever experienced. Outside the hospital room door, we could hear carolers singing "Joy to the World." It was the worst Christmas Eve I could imagine.

It seemed that the more I manipulated my body to become pregnant, the more elusive my baby became. My doctor discovered that I could not maintain a pregnancy because of fibroid tumors in my uterus. After four months of medication to shrink the tumors and then delicate major surgery to remove them, I could try again. The prospect of waiting six or seven months was almost unbearable.

I was depressed a lot during those months. Some mornings I would wake up at 4:00, feeling trapped in a black, airless box, my heart racing. I would cry uncontrollably, and had a hard time concentrating at work. I tried to figure out why this was happening to me. I had always believed that if you were a good person and did all the right things, your prayers would be answered. Now I came to believe that there were only two possible reasons why I wasn't getting pregnant: Either there was something wrong or bad about me and I was being punished, or it didn't matter whether you were good or not. The second explanation was too painful, so I chose to believe I had failed somehow and needed to turn into a good person before I could have my baby.

I had been raised a Catholic, but the church had long ago lost any meaning for me, partly because of its views of women. As a child, I loved to sit in a darkened church and watch the parade of priest and altar boys with their dangling pots of fragrant incense, holding the Eucharist to be blessed for Mass the following day. When I heard "Ave Maria" or smelled the incense or watched the pageantry, I felt I was part of something infinitely large and powerful and loving and sacred.

Month after month, I took fertility drugs, followed the protocol, and waited. All that happened was that I got more depressed. All the while, my husband continued to love me and to try to understand me, but he was approaching the end of his compassion. "A baby would be wonderful," he'd say. "But now can be wonderful, too. Why can't you see all you have? Why is this baby so important that nothing else has any meaning for you?"

One day, in a journal, I discovered a quote I had copied from a book written by a psychiatrist who lived in my town. The gist was that if you were willing to take the journey to find yourself, you'd always find a guide. I looked up the doctor in the phone book and made an appointment.

At the first session, the doctor took off his shoes, lit a candle, and asked me to describe what was going on with me here and now. I just crumbled and cried and cried with sadness, rage, helplessness. He prescribed Prozac because of the severity of my depression. Within days, my feelings of hopelessness lessened dramatically. I was still depressed, but I wasn't crying uncontrollably. I felt as though I'd come up for air after being underwater for a very long time.

I told the doctor I wanted him to help me change into a different, better person. He said he couldn't do that, and my heart fell. He said he could help me change into the person I already was. When I talked about fear, he told me about a two-headed snake. When I talked about loss of faith, he told me how eagles lay their eggs. When I talked about infertility, he told me that I needed to line my vessel. "You can't get nothing from nothing, Mol," he'd say. When I talked about unfairness, he'd say, "Shit happens and miracles happen."

Right. I didn't know what the hell he was talking about. But I listened, and gradually I began to hear. I heard stories and images about how you can strengthen yourself, about how to silence your ego so you can have a word with yourself. I began to notice the world differently. Like the moths, for example.

I arrived home one afternoon and found my carport wall covered with hundreds of large white moths. I had never seen anything like them before (and haven't seen them since). I called the county agricultural agent, who knew right away they were salt cedar marsh moths. He'd never heard of them in my part of town.

"How can I get rid of them?" I asked.

"Why do you have to get rid of them? They won't do you any harm. They'll die off naturally in a few weeks," he said.

"But there are so many of them. Will they eat my flowers? My stucco? The paint off our cars?"

76

"No," the agent said, "they don't eat anything during their entire adult lives, and they don't attract other critters. Just leave them alone. They're there to mate, but it's so late in the season I don't believe their eggs will take hold. Be patient; they'll be gone soon."

I let the moths stay where they were. Within three weeks, their numbers had dwindled to a handful. But their eggs held. Were they trying to tell me something? That, late in the season I, too, could lay an egg that held? No. More like, it's never too late in the season to take hold. What a pointless and narrow life I would lead if my whole adult existence centered on having a baby. These moths didn't eat, they didn't fly, they didn't do anything but mate in vain and cling to my wall and die. My God, could that happen to me? Gradually, I gave up waiting to see if I was pregnant each month and found other ways to feel joy.

I participated in an intensive weekend program for women. It was a pretty amazing weekend, even though I was so scared and guarded that I didn't participate as fully as I might have. Two powerful things stand out: making shields and the sweat lodge ceremony at dawn.

We were assigned to make our own personal shields, a decorative symbol of who we were and how we wanted to present ourselves to the world. Off I went into the surrounding forest, enjoying the beautiful day as I looked for twigs and flowers and pine cones and whatever else struck my fancy. Back at the house, I sat in a circle with the other women and made my shield, using paint and glitter and fabric and the twigs I had collected. It seemed I was just playing, putting something together out of odds and ends.

After my shield was finished, I looked at it closely and realized that all the twigs I had used had a bud at one end and a dead stump at the other. I immediately thought of life and death and how one follows the other, over and over. My life is inseparable from the lives of those I love and long to love, but it is my life and I will grow. Out of all the colors available, I'd used green and white. As I looked at the finished shield I knew it was my new spirit. Could this recently very depressed person really have made this? Every woman in the workshop found something in her shield that she needed to know. I still have my shield, and it still reminds me of growth, hope, and spirit.

The sweat lodge ceremony took place at dawn in a round enclosure made of wood frame and canvas cover. Twenty of us sat around a central pit filled with red hot rocks. Water was sprinkled on the rocks to create steam. In the blistering heat, afraid and uncomfortable, I was instructed to pray when my turn in the circle came around. The heat from the steam was searing, a woman was beating a drum outside, and suddenly I felt another heartbeat inside me. At that moment, I knew what "lining my vessel" meant. I had within me the capacity to feel the heartbeat of life even if I wasn't pregnant. Lining my vessel had to do with how many ways there are to feel full.

I had the same feeling I'd had as a child sitting in a darkened church listening to songs in Latin and smelling the candle wax and incense. I don't remember what I prayed about when my turn came, something about the kind of person I wanted to be. After four rounds of searing steam, it was over and I stood in the light of a new day.

From that day on, my life went on more evenly than it had. I still yearned for a child, but I was kinder to myself. I found a new doctor, a woman who was smart and kind and empathetic.

I enjoyed my life. I hiked and looked forward to weekend excursions. My husband and I took ballroom dancing lessons with friends, we entertained, we went out of town for weekends occasionally. I had fun.

And then my sister died. It was one of the horrors of my life. My family was racked with guilt and rage, and I became the vessel that helped sustain. In spite of my infertility, I had enough to nurture my loved ones. I had become stronger.

Four months after my sister's death, I again participated in a sweat lodge ceremony. The heat, the steam, the smells, the music, and the sense of community were overwhelming. This time, though, something inside me just let go. I had never experienced anything like it. I prayed, I cried, I came out of that ceremony feeling reborn. I didn't stop smiling for a week.

A few weeks later I was pregnant. And, true to form, within weeks I was bleeding. Back to bed for ten weeks. But this time was different. The first time I was on bedrest, I was tense and scared, waiting for the worst to happen. I didn't want any visitors because I looked like hell most of the time. I just wanted to hold that baby in at all costs. This time I was scared but more relaxed. I chose to trust that whatever happened, I could handle it. I welcomed some visitors. I tried my hand at watercolors. I read for fun, I read for inspiration. I wrote. But mostly, I tried to focus on the moment at hand and live it consciously.

The ten weeks passed, and we had made it through the first seventeen weeks. Hallelujah! I have never felt better in my life than I did during the last two trimesters of that pregnancy. There were days when I actually felt like I could shoot sparks from my fingertips. There were plenty of times when I was scared, but I never lost faith. I would survive, pregnant or not.

On September 13 at five minutes past midnight, we greeted our beautiful Sam. My baby is a precious gift, but that isn't the only reason I'd take this journey again. I've gained much more than just my son. It may sound trite, but instead of turning into someone else,

79

I learned to like being me. In the bargain, I found a way to trust life and live a meaningful life no matter what the external conditions might be. It's not that I'm deliriously happy all the time; I still get sad, I still get scared, and I know that there are things I'll just never understand. But I can let them go. Call me mom.

This is Molly's story. It's one of hope and participation. It's about healing ceremonies from psychotherapy to shield-making, women's groups and sweat lodges. In all of these events, we face our truth and find strength in community and believe that we can experience something special, like dreams coming true.

Telling the truth of one's story in a community of support that shares a common purpose has overwhelming potential for transformation. Set aside the time, create a sacred space where you can truly feel present in the moment, and you will experience something special—how dreams become possibilities.

AUTUMN
Late Adulthood (Ages 56–70)

House made of dusk

Vision dims at house's door

Still I see

Happily may I walk

With abundance may I walk

Happily may I walk

—from the Navajo

Nightway Chant

WHAT BECOMES OF us in these years? In our culture, these change-of-life years have become onerous ones. For many of us, becoming older means becoming undesirable, even ugly. Gray hair, less hair, wider hips, more wrinkles, slower reactions—our youth-obsessed culture assumes these things are the opposite of beauty. Menopause means not just giving up our procreative years, but also means loss of desire, attractiveness, and sexuality. In reality, like all seasons of life, this is a time of loss, and a time of growth. As Jung said it, "Aging people should know that their lives are not mounting and unfolding but that an inexorable inner process forces the contraction of life. For a young person it is almost a sin—and certainly a danger—to be too much occupied with himself; but for the aging person it is a duty and a necessity to give serious attention to himself.[1]

In men, the change of life is called the climacteric (from the Greek word meaning "critical"). It really is not the true equivalent of menopause. In menopause, a woman's level of the female hormone estrogen plunges sharply in a relatively short time, but men never undergo such a precipitous change in the concentration of the male hormonal equivalent, testosterone. Rather, it seems to decrease gradually from ages 45 to 70.[2,3] Carl explains:

> *Some of my colleagues think the male climacteric is a myth, but I felt my energies gradually begin to change in my late 40s. I went to bed earlier; the force of my urinary stream (which could once knock a paper cup off a picket fence) started dribbling. As a matter of fact, I couldn't do anything as fast as I once did. I had yet to learn that slow could also be good. I take some organic pills now. I swim instead of playing racquetball, I get a massage every week. I've learned how to breathe more slowly through daily Yoga.*
>
> *I've learned to appreciate going slowly, but that doesn't mean stopping. In fact, taking things at a slower pace can improve the experience. When I'm scuba diving I stay down twice as long now.*

Our culture is preoccupied with "fast"—from fast foods to one-hour photo developing, instantaneous communication (from satellites to car phones), computers, instant lottery winners, and instant highs with cocaine. In late adulthood, we discover that slow ain't bad. Slow means more time to experience pleasure in every moment. Time to sing songs, write poems, tell stories to somebody who wants to listen. Everybody's stories help us to look back and to make sense of our lives. They give us hope when we're down; they remind us to dare to dream.

Too often, however, autumn becomes the season of abandoned dreams. The daily drudgery of "taking care of business" has dulled them. Autumn ought to be the season in which we redefine ourselves; create a story that reveals our spirit. It is a time to review old habits, make some changes and see more clearly that tomorrow is *now*. Driven by inertia we sometimes tell ourselves lies until we get a heart attack or a divorce, or die.

The late adulthood transition can be especially difficult for a woman. Hormonally and culturally, menopause is often a defining point of passage in her life.[4,5] The only way to manage the stresses of this season is to look at it as a liberating, creative, reflective time for renewal. The ultimate goal of this season is to find new potentials that arrive with the freedom from physical reproduction and the rearing of children.

Our culture has no formal ceremony to mark a woman's transition from fecundity to infertility. Germaine Greer says that the lack of a rite of passage to mark the change, plus the sexual stereotyping of older women, has resulted in widespread despair among those undergoing this transition.[6] Depression can be avoided, or lessened, if you can make this a time to acquire new status and confidence. This article appeared recently in *The Arizona Daily Star:*[7]

Ruth Gardener of Tucson, 61, proudly identifies herself as a crone. But for Ruth, a retired nurse, the dictionary definition of crone as "an ugly, withered old woman, a hag" doesn't quite make it. She sees a crone as a woman of wisdom and experience with traditions to pass along from generation to generation.

Ruth celebrated being a crone through a croning ceremony. There are no established rules for croning ceremonies. They can be as individual as the women who create and take part in them.

Ruth spent a long time planning her ceremony. When the time came, many older women gathered to be croned, and their daughters "came from far and wide and did the ritual." Their ceremony took place in the desert before an altar covered with purple, the color of the crone. On it were placed pictures of the mothers along with symbolic objects—things that were important to them or that they had made or seen or done. There were also candles, salt, bread, fruit, flowers, and water. In the ceremony, one of the daughters said, "You have lived long and have many earthly years of experience." After singing and drumming and dancing, the daughters placed flowered crowns upon their mothers' heads.

Said one of the newly croned women, "If I had carried through my life all of the understanding and wisdom that I now have at fifty-six, I'm sure I would have been a better parent, a better woman, a better everything."

Storytelling, ceremony, and passing the family history from one generation to the next are important parts of all croning ceremonies. A growing number of women from 40 to 90 years old are celebrating their age through these ceremonies, announcing not only their acceptance but their enjoyment of their aging.

We are clearly living in a time when people feel the void left by the absence of initiation ceremonies in their lives.

Furthermore, our culture maintains its images through slick advertising and hard-sell commercialism. That's how we get a picture of who we are supposed to be. Too often, that cultural stereotype means someone over 50 is no longer productive or beautiful. These cultural images present obstacles to the true work of late adulthood: passing beyond the biological role of reproduction and moving into the spiritual world.

For many Native American tribes, autumn is a woman's time of greatest power. At menopause, she breaks free of the routine and disappears for a while in order to reflect on her new role as wisdom-keeper. In Indian country, from the time a woman bleeds for the first time until her last period, she gathers with other women every month in a ceremony to celebrate the gift that brings life to earth. Carl's wife, Elaine, explains what happened to her during her menopause:

It began when I asked my husband to please move the air conditioning vent slats in the bedroom. He said we'd been sleeping in the same bed in the same location for twenty years. Maybe it wasn't the air conditioning. I insisted it was getting hotter at night. Then the daytime sweats started, and I understood what hot flashes were. But I was too young, strong, and mentally fit to be so powerfully affected by these hormonal surges and emotional outbursts when I got trapped in a bitchy mood.

I thought I'd go through menopause just the way my mother and mother-in-law and other women of their generation had done. No fuss, no discussion, no problem, as if they'd had some kind of magical hysterectomy that made their periods stop one day, and then it was all over.

My gynecologist of sixteen years explained my symptoms and prescribed hormonal replacement therapy. I struggled over whether to take the hormones, they might increase the risk of cancer, but if I didn't take them, I could get osteoporosis or heart disease. Finally I took them, but when I went off the pills for the last five days of the cycle I got excruciating headaches. I phoned my gynecologist, who told me to see a neurologist to be sure I didn't have a brain tumor. I was shocked. "I can't believe that's your first response to these symptoms," I said, but he had already hung up.

I found another doctor who understood that menopause is an exceptional time in a woman's whole life, not just in her pelvis. She suggested I see a nutritionist, an herbalist, and a massage therapist. They all helped. But underneath it all I kept telling myself, get over this already, your body just doesn't fail like this, get back in control.

Instinctively, I think, I knew that my search had to become more spiritual, that I had to look someplace besides doctors to find the strength to deal with my intense symptoms. Not quite knowing why, I decided to accompany my husband to a Lakota Sundance ceremony.

If a woman has her period, her "moon time," during the Sundance, she goes to a separate place called the Moon Lodge. She can't go to the arbor where the Sundance is held or prepare food in the communal kitchen. So awesome is women's power at this time that they could affect the men dancing inside, just by their closeness.

I didn't know any of this when I got there, I only knew that on the first day of Sundance I got my first period in six months. I thought, "Just my luck, now I won't even be able to see the dance." I didn't want to go away to a separate place. I had no idea what was expected of me, and I was afraid to be alone with strangers. But in spite of my fear, I sensed that the experience might help me in my struggle with this season. I packed my necessities, a sleeping bag, a change of clothing, some reading material, and off I went.

The Moon Lodge consisted of several tents, with folding chairs, mats, blankets, and sleeping bags everywhere. Food and water were available under a communal tarp. These women I didn't know saw me with my bundle and greeted me like a long-lost sister. When I arrived, ten or eleven women were holding a Talking Circle. I was certain I was the oldest woman there.

Each greeted me, as they moved clockwise around the circle and made room for me to sit. Each woman spoke in turn while holding an eagle feather, a gift from one of the Sundancers. Everyone talked about what it was like to be a woman at this time in her life. We'd been brought together at this moment because we were all on our moon, because we were women. From the 12-year-old, to me at 50, we came together in this sacred place to gain strength from our womanness. We talked about child abuse, sexual abuse, marriage, children, hopes, fears, even menopause. And we heard each other. I felt respected, appreciated, even honored, as an older woman with some wisdom to share from having made it this far. I felt wonderful! The whole community considered us special, and the encampment looked to us as powerful people—not outcasts, just powerful.

People brought us food, families came to visit us, and then they left. While in the Moon Lodge, women participated in a Talking Circle every day. Some left, others joined us to be part of our special womanness.

They called me Grandmother, and they meant that I was a woman of wisdom. When my turn came to leave, I didn't want to leave. I felt so good, enriched, and proud. I also felt jealous that my culture didn't provide such an experience for my daughters, my sister, my friends. From the moment I left that circle I knew in my heart, at some spiritual core, that I was empowered in a different way.

I still participate in women's healing circles. We laugh, we commiserate, we cope, but most important, we come together as individuals with power. This is the abiding gift; this time is a seasonal gift of new awakening. Today I look differently at my symptoms; I see myself more as a creature of beauty than one who suffers.

A crucial aspect of ceremonies is the involvement of others. As a species, human beings need each other. It is through relationships of mutuality, of shared interest, by giving and getting, that we find what we wish to gain. Whether it's an Alcoholics Anonymous meeting, a bereavement group, or a Native American Talking Circle, connecting with people helps us achieve our innermost strivings. Once we have been joined in a community, we take a little piece of that community with us when we move on.

We create community when we come together to make sense of our realities by beginning to share our lives, our stories, and the wisdom we have acquired. Renewing and sharing our spirit selves and the truth of who we are is the path of fulfillment in the season of autumn.

EARLY WINTER
Aging (Ages 71–85)

House made of evening light
Happily may I walk
Happily with abundant showers may I walk
Happily with abundant plants may I walk
Happily on the trail of pollen may I walk
Happily may I walk
—from the Navajo Nightway Chant

OLD AGE, WHEN we retire from the busyness of adulthood, is the time to share abundance and wisdom, to tell the stories we've accumulated. Our 70s are the time to become an elder, to share what we've acquired with others who are ready to receive it.[1]

As one approaches the elder years, a powerful ceremony is the writing of an ethical will. By this time of life, you probably have prepared a legal will and made arrangements to take care of your affairs once you are gone. The purpose of the ethical will is different; it is a way to define your deepest values, beliefs, and instructions for living a good life.[2] Use it to share what's important to you with your family. Talk to the grandchildren about it, make a videotape, or write an autobiography. Use it to tell the story about what's important to you, what you've learned that has made a difference in your life. It will connect you with future generations in a joyful way. Don't wait until it's too late. When Howard's father passed away suddenly, Howard was given an unexpected and priceless gift:

After my father's unexpected death, my mother went into their study and retrieved a stack of papers. She explained that my father had been working on something just before he died and had seemed unusually pleased to have finished it. As I scanned the yellow lined paper, the first thing I noticed was his peculiar handwriting—he had always printed and had never written in cursive. Tears filled my eyes as I read over this document entitled "Ethical Will of Dave Silverman." It was a short yet beautiful distillation of everything my father had learned during his life, everything he valued in life. The last paragraph read:

By the time you read this ethical will, I no longer will be with you physically. I will have departed this earth as have all the generations before me. I don't think I should be continually mourned, since this is God's plan and departing physically is his destiny for all of us. I would be happy if I would be remembered by you and the future generations of our family rather than being continuously mourned. Hoping where I'll be will give me that position of being able to look down on all of you from the life hereafter. I am sure I will be able to see you and my descendants, smile and beam about all of you who remain on this earth.

The next night, as friends and family gathered for a brief prayer service at my mother's home, I read my father's ethical will to all *present. Afterward, nobody was able to utter a word. What an incredible comfort. What an incredible blessing. What an incredible father.*

What does it mean to become an elder? Your own ideas about being older have been formed from experiences with your grandparents, your teachers, the media. Increasingly, our culture offers negative images that diminish the power of the elder. We don't pay much attention to the process of being an elder anymore. Nobody has the time to listen, so it's hard to find an audience that will hear our stories. Some will seek you out, though—talk to them about whatever wisdom you've accumulated; it needs to be shared. Your experience is a source of abundance that can enrich lives. If you keep it to yourself, you lose its power. Ours is a culture that acquires things and holds onto them—objects, land, even outer space is owned, marketed, and sold. The planet gets bartered like a commodity, not revered like a sacred entity that sustains our lives. Our culture seduces its younger members into the belief that ownership is the only way you can get control of something. You think you can have control of it, when the truth is that it's got you. Sharing abundance, rather than accumulating it, is what keeps us healthy.

In Indian country, people celebrate this season of aliveness by giving things away, thereby saying, "Thank you for my life." Among the Northwest Coastal Indian tribes, the concept of giveaway once held a central place in ceremonial life. Once someone had accumulated as much as he could, in esteem, stature, and material goods, he was expected to give it away in ceremonies called potlatches.

The word "potlatch" comes from the Nootka word "pat-shatl," which means "giving." Potlatch was the ultimate celebration of life. It was in the giveaway that the Salish and other tribes set in motion the harmony that would replenish them and the earth. The Salish knew that they could never run out of things necessary for life as long as the tide came in and out.

When the white man came, he saw this ceremony as debauched and wasteful, so potlatches were outlawed by the federal government in the early 1900s. The new culture enforced its code by requiring people to surrender their ceremonial regalia. Without ceremonies to transmit its values, tribal life was threatened. Tribes began to quarrel among themselves; they fought about who was keeping more for themselves.

Some refused to surrender and hid their costumes, masks, drums, and rattles and stayed connected to the spirit of things. The potlatches were celebrated "underground." These rebels understood that without their ceremonies they would not be able to appreciate their unique place in the universe. Today, those tribes who remember their songs are clamoring to get their regalia back from museums around the world. The tribes are alive, and their instruments need to be used.

In potlatches being celebrated up and down the Northwest Coast today, the elders are teaching the language, dances, and songs, even recreating ceremonial objects in school workshops. The young people treasure these gifts that remind them of who they are. The elders say the return to ceremony is a reminder of the power of prophecy and prayer.

We all acquire ceremonial objects during our lifetimes.

Eventually, there comes a time to let them go as well, as this story of Carl's patient Vincent illustrates:

For thirty years, Vincent worked as a manager in the automobile business, saving $200 a month, which he compounded in a money-market account. He had figured out how much it would take to sustain him and his wife, Christina, in retirement. They planned to spend their "golden years" in a travel trailer, fly fishing in every blue-ribbon trout stream in North America. Christina was an artist who painted miniature animals on porcelain charms, which she sold at craft fairs. Her dream was to travel to wilderness areas and see firsthand all those animals that were the source of her inspiration. This shared dream sustained them during the hard times in their lives.

But, like most plans, this one had to be modified. The pundits say life is what happens to you while you're busy making other plans. Neither Vincent nor Christina anticipated that she would die of a heart attack at age 64, one year before their journey into old age was to have begun.

At the loss of his partner and his dream, Vincent gave up. He'd sit and stare into space; he didn't wash, shave, or change his clothes. His only son, a hospital pharmacist, called me one day to ask what he should do about his dad, who was becoming more uncommunicative and regressed. I told him that profound depression in response to a major loss was not uncommon, but it's good to deal with it sooner rather than later because the longer the symptoms last, the harder they are to get rid of.

When he became unresponsive and started drooling, he was hospitalized. Drug therapy did not have much of an effect on him. He began to soil himself and continued to lose weight. They decided to try electroconvulsive therapy, which had had miraculous results. By the second treatment he had begun to brighten. He fed himself, showered, and by the end of a month he was participating in groups.

But improvement came with a price. His short-term memory was impaired by the treatments. He couldn't keep track of what he ate for breakfast, but he could remember the name of his sixth-grade teacher. However, he could still tie fishing flies, and he was now sustaining himself.

Vincent hadn't talked about himself much. One day in group, he began to describe, in exquisite detail, the streams in which he had fished as a boy. In our sessions together, he told me what flies worked best, where, and at what time of day. He said he could teach me to tie them. I ought to try it, he said. Why not? I like to go fishing. So he had his son bring in his fly-tying equipment. That's what we did for the next month. He'd show me the feathers and where they came from, then clamp a hook into the miniature vise and wrap it all up. Each fly had its own story about how it got its name, when and where to use it. I liked listening to his stories, and it brought him out in such animated ways.

One afternoon another patient, seeing us at work, asked Vincent if he could watch. That's how fly-tying got started in the hospital. Other patients heard about it, and it became a class. Through sharing what he knew and loved, Vincent began connecting with others. He started talking about his wife, and one day he began to think about what he was going to do with the rest of his life.

After three months in the hospital, Vincent was discharged.

He sold his house soon and bought a motor home. In the beginning he fished and camped alone. We corresponded, so I asked him to visit a colleague of mine who consulted at a senior citizen center in Boise. I told my friend about the class Vincent taught at the hospital, and he thought it might work at his place, too. He asked

Vincent if he'd teach some fly-tying at the center, and Vincent taught at the center a couple of times a week for about a month. From there it spread. Vincent went to fish in Wyoming, where my friend happened to know someone in Cheyenne, and he taught fly-tying there. Soon, he had referrals almost every place on his route. From Alaska to Arizona he spent a year traveling, chasing good weather and good fishing, and teaching old people how to tie flies.

Some people, those with whom he became very fond, he took fishing with him. To them he gave a porcelain pin or pendant that his wife had made. He told these people Christina's story. "She would have appreciated this time and place," he'd say. In this way, he felt they were sharing their dream together. He brought her to every place he went, and gave it all away.

By giving his knowledge of fly fishing and by giving his wife's creations, Vincent enriched his life as well as the lives of others. Winter isn't a time for holding on, but for giving away. Winter is the time for inner growth, and this growth has nothing to do with digging in—it has to do with surrendering.

A friend of Carl's told him this story:

The Reverend stood with friends and family around the hospital bed of a 70-year-old man who had convinced them it was time to end his kidney dialysis treatments. He was never one who liked dependency and had always called the shots in his life. Knowing his wishes, his family withdrew medical treatments and decided to hold a ceremony. Since there is no specific service for terminating life support in the Episcopal Book of Common Prayer, the Reverend chose to adapt the

Communion, the calling of awareness of Christ within us and within each other.

Knowing his hours were numbered, they all held hands, shared Communion, and told each other of their love. In his dying, they saw the proud and determined man of faith he had always been in life. He died peacefully that night.

The essence of who we are, our spirit, needs to be shared. People who connect in this way share a vision that leaves each of them feeling better. Just as important, they pass along wisdom fragments that can help younger relatives prepare for their elderhood.

There is always someone to share with. There are a multitude of ways of sharing. In a program called Time Dollars, people give their time, their most precious commodity, to elderly and incapacitated persons.[3] Participants might go shopping for somebody, clean a bathroom, drive Aunt Millie to her doctor's appointment, or pick up Tom and take him to a church service. The time each person gives is "banked," and the giver can receive that amount of time from somebody else if she or he ever needs it. A bank president who wouldn't mow your lawn for a thousand dollars will do it for nothing. Someday, someone will be available to help him out.

If we're going to survive old age, our attitude and how we feel are more important than what we know or what we own. Several authors stress a positive approach to life as the key to strengthening the body and the mind.[4,5,6] Our immune function, which guards our bodies against disease, responds to positive emotions such as altruism, compassion, and co-operation. It's been said so many times that it has become a cliche, but by giving, we receive more than we give.

Connecting our hearts and souls, making relationships, and sharing openly can protect our health. Researchers have found that heart patients who are connected in an intimate relationship, whether with a spouse, a close friend, or a pet, are three times more likely to survive for five years than those who aren't. Conversely, isolation and loneliness lead to higher mortality. Men isolate themselves more frequently than women as they age, and men also suffer significantly higher death rates.[7,8]

We can tie into this season by giving away what we have cherished and nurtured for all these years—even if it is simply our wisdom. A wise man said that the only things we take with us are what we leave behind. Don't save it for a final bash—give it away. We need to tell our stories to the next generation to help them make sense of their lives.

LATE WINTER
Old Age (Ages 85+)

House made of evening light

Happily may I walk

Happily with abundant showers may I walk

Happily with abundant plants may I walk

Happily on the trail of pollen may I walk

Happily may I walk

—from the Navajo Nightway Chant

IS THE AGE you'll reach genetically preordained? To some extent, the answer is yes—genes do matter. One of the best ways to live to a ripe old age is to have long-lived ancestors. Add to that a healthy lifestyle, and you've got a lot of bases covered. No matter what the life span of your ancestors, at least this much is clear: As a species, we are programmed to survive long past the end of our reproductive periods—well into the 80s and beyond. Because of this longevity, society needs to expand its thinking about aging, because we are going to experience breathtaking increases in life span in our own lifetimes.[1]

Many people now face the challenge of living into their ninth or tenth decades. The task of this season is to feel as good as you can and to treasure every day. Physician and researcher Deepak Chopra suggests the cultivation of positive factors that can influence and even retard aging, such as a satisfying job, a happy long-term relationship, personal gratification, and a regular daily work routine.[2]

In late winter, enjoy the vibrancy of life. Stop worrying. Addressing this task does not mean denying your arthritic pains, disabilities, or insecurities. It simply means that it would be better to come to every day with joy, saying thank you.

This season is almost like being a teenager again. It's a season of anticipation, fear, isolation. Yet we still feel quite together. Doris Noyes was 89 years old when she wrote this for *Newsweek* in September 1994.

One glance and you'd know I'm a Senior. The hair on my head is white, and although my face is not overly lined, it's obvious. While I work at standing erect, my shoulders slouch a bit. And, despite regular swim sessions and frequent brisk walks, I have difficulty hiding my protruding belly. But the inner me, the emotional me, is so frequently a teener. I feel much as I did 75 years ago: alone, tremulous and fearful about my future.

Were Charles Darwin to arise from the dead, I'd say to him, "There's a new subspecies abroad today, sir." And I'd tell him about its evolution during the latter part of the twentieth century when humankind—particularly womankind—was living longer and longer in an amazing state of physical health. But I'd have to come clean as to the emotional downside; the sense of queasiness that from time to time overtakes an otherwise reasonably fit body. For today I'm often jittery and "out of it" as in long-ago days—no special boyfriend

or agemates. Three husbands have predeceased me, and my longtime
female intimates have also made their final exits.

Obviously seniors are not teeners. The journey now is
mostly downhill. Too many people look at them as self-
absorbed and objects of disdain (much the same as we view
adolescents). In spite of their eccentricities, our elders have
something to teach us; they are a treasure trove of stories
and experience.

The task of old age is to come to each day saying,
"Thank you." When being alive is no longer sufficient to keep
you believing that life is good, your spirit flags, and if it's
flagging for too long, your spirit will be gone.

When a star collapses, all the fuel at its core, gasses and
fissionable material, burns up, and the star implodes. The
crust collapses, and there's a massive explosion whose flash
can be seen ten million light-years away. The supernova is
the brightest light in the night sky, and then it's gone. This
is how it is with us. For a brief time, we light up the night
sky and then we're gone. We will go sooner if we let our
inner fuel burn up. The human spirit is that inner fuel—it's
what sparks our lives. Some people abandon their indomi-
table spirits because they do not wish to fight for their lives.

Times of transition are always times of opportunity.
Times to develop mastery in a confrontation with an unfa-
miliar world. The downside is that times of transition are also
times of threat, because they force a confrontation with the
old established order. If you do not come to transitions, particularly at the end of life, feeling the inner force of your
spirit, then you set yourself up for grief. Without an indom-

itable spirit, the passage through which we move in life becomes very constricted.

Sooner or later, you realize that there's an end to "becoming". All of the pop psychological rhetoric about becoming all you can be, forever, doesn't change the ultimate realization that one day life's journey will be over. How do we face the fact that all of us are mortal and still be able to enjoy our moments? Carl helped his friend Joyce with a ceremony:

I was in Chicago, and the evening before my lecture I visited a friend who was living with an inoperable brain tumor. The year before, Joyce had developed double vision; examination revealed a rare brain tumor that was destroying the brain at the base of her skull. The tumor was fast-growing, so her doctors tried to relieve the pressure inside her skull by suctioning some of it out. Unfortunately, they had to abbreviate the procedure because she bled profusely. Surgery was followed with proton beam radiation, a new experimental procedure that yielded some improvement. Within nine months, Joyce began to have hoarseness in her throat and difficulty in swallowing. Her mental faculties remained intact, and she was still working regularly as a nurse. Repeated brain scans revealed the tumor was growing, but surgery was very risky because technically the procedure was very difficult. But if they didn't operate, she would soon be blind, unable to walk or even breathe on her own. Joyce knew that she could die on the table, but she also knew that she didn't want to become immobilized or incompetent. "It isn't worth being alive," she said. She was told that with surgery she might have two good years, but ultimately the tumor would grow again.

I saw her two weeks before her anticipated surgery. Over dinner she talked about her feeling that she would not survive the operation.

I asked why she decided to have surgery if it really wasn't what she wanted to do. She outlined all her reasons again. I suggested if she had decided to do it, why not come to it with positivity, hope, even joy at the possibility of a couple more good years? I then suggested that we create a little ceremony to send her off to surgery. I told her about the family hair-washing ceremony and described the people walking back and forth from the bathroom to carry in pitchers of warm water, and the music and incense. Joyce loved the thought and said a washing ritual was perfect for her. She was the wife of an ordained minister; both she and her husband were leaders in their spiritual community. The ceremony could help her wash away her doubts, she said. She called the children, told them she would like to do something special the night before surgery, and asked each of them to bring a memento of themselves that she could keep with her while she was in the hospital.

I said good-bye and the next morning I took a drive up the shore of Lake Michigan. Quite by accident I came upon an ornate temple that overlooked the lake. It looked like a cake decoration spun from ribbon candy. I stopped to look at it more closely; it turned out to be the main house of Baha'i worship in northern America. As I walked up to it, I couldn't tell where the entrance was. A circular structure, there was no front or back. The entire temple was surrounded by marble steps, and you could enter it from any direction. Inside the sanctuary, the chairs were arranged in a circle; there was no pulpit. On one side facing the lake was a small podium with a light and microphone where a member of the congregation, the Reader, would read from the writings of the Prophet Baha'u'llah. One in a line of prophets that extends from Buddha, Moses, Jesus, Mohammed, Gandhi, Wallenberg and King, Baha'u'llah appeared on the planet one hundred and fifty years ago and preached that the Earth was one community and that all mankind were its citizens. He emphasized that all of the prophets that ever appeared on the Earth have proclaimed the same faith.

This information was summarized in the visitor center in the temple basement and reminded me of Thoreau's words, that a true disciple is someone who can see another's God as his own.

I sat down in the center of the sanctuary and dropped my head back to look at the incredibly intricate design on the domed ceiling. In the middle was an inscription written in Arabic calligraphy that read, "Oh Thou, the glory of the most glorious." I stared at the ceiling, while the noon sun flashed like a strobe through the grillwork, until the design began to move into a whirling mandala. In the middle I saw Joyce's face smiling at me. It is our connections that succor us in this world. This is what life is all about. In getting nearer to each other, we get closer to hope. In the Baha'i temple I prayed for Joyce's recovery: "May you thrive in this world. May the four winds blow you safely home and may I remember you in the world to come."

After her surgery, I received a package in the mail that contained these cards and letters.

Dear Carl,

Your unexpected visit began a series of surprising events. It provided me with a positive view of what had been, to me, a questionable behavior. The fact that your visit to our home was enjoyable for you, personally, as well as for Larry and me, was a tremendous affirmation. The meditation, during which I pictured empowering the surgeon to remove the tumor, has left a powerful and lasting attitude change. For the first time I can picture life after the surgery.

Another helpful result of your visit was your suggestion that I have my children and I share a ritual while they were here. This turned out to be a very meaningful evening. I did ask both my son and daughter, Wayne and Peggy, to bring gifts that I could take to the hospital. Peggy brought a storyteller figure, and Wayne brought a handmade statue reflecting what he does at work. During our time together, Peggy washed my hair and Wayne washed my feet. Both experiences were deeply touching and energizing, physically and emotionally. I saw a side of my son which he usually does not show. He was gentle, patient, and tender. I shared a list I had written about both of them which told of their positive character strengths. I also shared with them the things I had learned about myself in the last few weeks, which included insights gained during your visit, and at my unit farewell party. It turned out to be a very warm and bonding experience for our whole family.

At my unit party, I was telling my nursing peers about your visit. My supervisor seemed to have a revelation. She called for her purse and handed me the keys to the hospital unit, which I had returned to her earlier that evening. She said I was to keep the keys. In my experience at the hospital, I have never known anyone to be allowed to keep their keys after they quit. It was very moving. The rest of the evening, I heard from these friends and co-workers, ways I had contributed to them, personally, and the children we worked with (on the Child and Adolescent Psychiatric Unit). The next day, during an opportunity for reflection, I felt that for the first time, I understood who I really am. Your visit and the unit party resulted in a life-giving experience for me, a sense of how much I am loved.

Thank you so much for visiting us and for all the positive contributions you have made in my life. I feel a new sense of empowerment as I enter the hospital tomorrow.

God bless you. Much love,

Joyce

P.S. I am enclosing some meaningful and healing messages which Peggy brought me. These are a sample (for you to keep) of 28 uplifting cards I received, created for me by her fourth graders.

Attached to another letter with a Post-It sticker was this note:

This is my sister's beautiful response to your suggestion that family members send things.

Dear Joyce,

When you asked for something that would remind you of us and our relationship, I thought a long time and couldn't help but think of the time the three of us were making up animal characters to fit our individual traits. It all started when I was being very stubborn about something and we started calling me the mule. We decided we should all have an animal we could relate to, so we decided you should be the bear because of your strength. Shirley was the fox for her ability to plan and think before she acted. I talked to Shirley and we thought that we should send small replicas of these animals. Hopefully, they will bring you something of us and also the characteristics of the animals they represent. May you become as stubborn as the mule as you are in surgery. May this characteristic help you fight with all you have to come through and stay with us. May you be as strong as the bear so that your strength may be multiplied and keep you safe against all odds. May the fox make you cunning and give you the presence of mind to ask the right questions and to prepare with care and thoughtfulness.

Keep them close, and may they bring you close to us and the strength of all their characteristics combined.

Love,

Phyllis

Joyce included a third letter with a Post-It note saying, *This is from my daughter:*

Dear Dr. Hammerschlag,

My mom asked me to write and tell you about our time, when we observed the family ritual together. At first I wasn't sure if we were going to be able to pull my brother away from his T.V. show but when we said this is the time Mom wants us to do something special together, he became very agreeable. We started by washing my mom's hair. My brother, Wayne, jumped in and helped hold her neck up so she would be more comfortable as he was leaning over the sink. Wayne asked if there was some special music she might enjoy in the background. (Smart guy! Great idea!) That lent an even more special atmosphere to our time. My dad cried as he let my brother and me do the physical work. He was touched by the love the two of us were displaying. Then my brother said that since I had washed mom's hair (he did a lot of the work in this), it would probably be pleasant for her to have her feet washed, and he did that. He was very attentive to details like was the water the correct temperature, etc. I was amazed. Also, Wayne never asked why we were doing these things, just the fact that we were sharing a special family time before Mom's surgery seemed to be enough for him.

Then, my mom talked to us about what had been going on in her life the past few weeks and she read a list of our positive traits as she had observed them (relating stories from our youth as well as present day observations). My brother continued to massage my mom's feet. My mom had already opened Wayne's gift as she brought it out and opened those she had received from me and her sister. It was a very comfortable and close time of sharing for us. Thank you for stopping in to see my parents. It made an incredible difference in my mom's pre-surgery attitude! She called me after you had been there.

106

The change in her outlook had become positive, hopeful and much more peaceful. It was a blessing to all of us to have her able to approach her surgery with this more assured outlook. As I sit here in the hospital, the day before her surgery, with all these preparatory procedures being imposed upon her, I am so glad that my mom is approaching this knowing that she is loved *and* valued.

What a ceremony!

Paul Brinkley-Rogers, a friend of Carl's who writes features for the *Arizona Republic*, is old as reporters go. He's from the reportorial school that tells the story behind the story, not just the apparent facts. Here's what happened to him driving out in the desert one afternoon just to see what was out there.

I happened on two old women looking under the hood of their ancient Dodge. So I slowed down and got out of my pickup truck and offered to help. They told me they only had $5 and knew their prospects of being found weren't good until I miraculously discovered them.

They'd come to this isolated place looking for desert wildflowers. Clara was 85, her friend Lizzie was 87. They were retired schoolteachers who had been together for over forty years. They were driving a 1968 Dodge they had bought new in Kansas City more than twenty years ago.

While Lizzie was under the hood banging on the carburetor, Clara told me that her friend was facing a terminal illness. "She won't last long," Clara said, "just like those wildflowers out there in the desert. That's why she comes out here every day, looking up and down the dirt roads in these Vulture Mountains." Since it was the dry season, they'd been lucky to see even a few of the desert lupines and the brilliant paintbrush that made the desert come alive.

Later Lizzie told me that the doctor in Phoenix said she had only a month to live. "I've got cancer of someplace or another that I don't even care to remember," she said, "but I sure would like to see the lupines bloom." She knew it might be too late in the season, but she had to keep looking. She never knew what she'd see and she wanted to see it all, that day.

When they finished working on the car, Lizzie banged the solenoid casing with a hammer, cussing sometimes, pleading at others, and told Clara to turn the ignition. Nothing happened, so Lizzie whacked it a second time, cussing, and Clara said to me, "Don't mind what she's saying." Just then the ancient V-8 engine burst into life. While Lizzie was putting her tools away in the trunk, Clara pulled out a letter Lizzie had written her and read it to me. It said, "Thank you for being my pal all these years. When I'm gone, I want you to take my ashes out to the wildflowers. You don't have to tell anybody, it's just between you and me. Scatter me where you can see me, scatter me in the spring when every day brings the most beautiful flowers I have ever seen."

Scattering ashes among the flowers, washing feet, and creating sacred amulets are some of the ceremonies of healing that sustain us. In Indian country they say there is no life line; rather, it's a life spiral. All Native American life symbols are circular. From the time we emerge on this road of life, we move with the sun. When it sets, that ending yields a new beginning. Beginnings are always a place beyond our current awareness. At this age, we can't wait around for either beginnings or endings, but we can be positive, joyful and thankful.

THE DEATH TRANSITION

With beauty may I walk

With beauty before me may I walk

With beauty behind me may I walk

With beauty below me may I walk

With beauty above me may I walk

With beauty all around me may I walk

In beauty it is finished

In beauty it is finished

—from the Navajo Nightway Chant

AT LAST COMES the time of letting go. The sun, having traveled from its source of emergence in the east, goes toward its final passing in the west. As we usher in the darkness, we are reminded that all existence follows this pattern of creation. Everything comes and everything goes. Sometimes the mission of a soul can find completion through the use of symbolism.

Some people are surprised that, even when they are faced with death, ceremonies can help fulfill dreams. It is particularly powerful to use ceremonies to begin preparing for the death transition, for the one dying and even more so for the survivors. The "work" of ceremony is bringing people together for a common purpose, and this helps us rally.

The end of life is the time for return. Among the Hasidim who flourished in eastern Europe in the eighteenth and nineteenth centuries, experiencing a "conscious" death was a very high aspiration. Close disciples would gather at the deathbeds of their masters, hoping to receive their final and ultimate expressions of faith and wisdom. Many stories of these events bear powerful witness to the unique character of the individual:

> His disciples came to visit Rabbi Eliezer as he lay ill. They said, "Master, teach us the paths by which we may attain eternal life." He replied, "Show concern for the honor of your friends; set your children at the feet of the wise, who will keep them from idle thoughts; and, when you pray, know before Whom you stand. Thus will you win eternal life."

The end of life is a time for feeling the power of prayer. Even if you have prayed before, prayer acquires a different significance as you prepare to let go. It becomes the only thing left, as the physical body and the possessions of this life deteriorate. Prayer is a path on the search for answers to the big existential questions: Who am I, why am I here, what will happen to me after I die?

On this final journey to the spirit world, you look at what you once thought was important and wonder what part it has in your life now. This is a time for experiencing beauty, mystery, and awe, as Albert Einstein explains: "The most beautiful thing we can experience is the mysterious. It is the source of all true art and science."[1] Some of us are fortunate enough to learn these lessons earlier in life. Here is what Carl experienced:[2]

I once believed that the most important task in life was to explain its mysteries. Everything had answers if we could just ask the right questions. Science and rationality held the promise for civilization's fulfillment. That was what I believed until I met Bill Dalton, an old Hopi medicine man, whose Indian name was Soloho. He taught me that not every question has an answer and that the lack of an answer does not mean that the question is not important to ask.

I visited him regularly for more than a decade during my monthly flights to the reservation. He and his Apache wife lived in a small shack near Ft. Apache. I'd eat lunch with him every month while he talked about herbs and natural medicines. I knew nothing about herbs, although I liked them in my food. Distinguishing a carrot plant from a radish leaf exceeds my capacity, but Soloho had a relationship with these plants. He felt the essence of their unique powers and could recognize them by leaf, bark, root, and smell.

He also liked asking me riddles. Why does a mountain lion have a bushy tail? Why is it that beetles never look up? In all our years together, I could never answer one of his riddles. I tried to prepare myself by studying trivia books or memorizing obscure facts from the fillers in the Sunday New York Times. *But I never answered one. In my frustration, I finally insisted that he explain why he continued to torment me with questions I could not answer. His answer came in the form of a story.*

Soloho once treated a well-known singer in Hawaii who, for some reason, had been unable to perform. After he "worked on" him, he was able to go on stage that night. The story was published in the local paper, and some kahunas (native Hawaiian healers) invited Soloho to attend a ceremony.

Not knowing what to expect, Soloho went to the location. The kahunas blindfolded him and eventually led him up a mountainside into a cave where the blindfold was removed. Soloho saw that he had crawled through a narrow passage leading into a chamber. In the middle of the cavern was a sunken pool into which steps had been carved. The kahunas chanted and moved their arms, just as Hopis do in certain ceremonies. The head kahuna took Soloho to the pool's edge and asked him to look at the water and tell what he saw.

Soloho said he saw ripples that appeared almost as waves on the water's surface. The kahuna asked him to explain their presence. So-loho knew that he saw waves, that the waves were there, but he knew the mountain wasn't moving and that he was higher than sea level. He didn't know why there were waves, but he knew the kahuna had asked him an important question. So he answered: "I don't know why there are waves but I know they are important."

The head kahuna nodded and got undressed, motioning Soloho to do so as well. They both walked down the stairs into the pool. Soloho's initiation was complete.

The riddle still escaped me, so I asked Soloho what the answer was. He laughed and said, "You white people are all the same. What's the answer? The kahunas didn't know the answer either. All they know is that when the waves stop, civilization will come to an end." Some questions don't have answers, it's enough to know that they are important.

That same message is in Torah, the Koran, the King James Bible, and cave-wall drawings. Recognize the importance of the questions, but accept the mystery of what cannot be known.

As death approaches, we must deal with our growing uncertainty. All the information we have thus far acquired does not answer the questions we face at the end. Our science falls short when we seek certainty about the purpose and meaning of our lives. Genuine answers require a leap of faith.

When he was about to die from cancer at age 69, Richard Feynman, arguably the most brilliant scientist since Einstein, said:

> I can live with doubt and uncertainty. I think it's more interesting to live not knowing than to have answers that might be wrong. I have approximate answers and possible beliefs and different degrees of certainty about different things, but I'm not absolutely sure of anything and there are many things I don't know anything about, such as whether it means anything to ask why we're here.[3]

Whenever our end comes, it gets clearer that the final destination is not something we know a lot about. We can learn from some people who have seen a glimpse of what's beyond.

Raymond Moody, a thanatologist and best-selling author, has reported hundreds of case histories of people who have experienced clinical death and then survived.[4,5] Descriptions of near-death experiences seem to have several common themes: floating above one's body, a feeling of serenity, seeing light at the end of a tunnel, or seeing one's dead relatives.[6,7]

Some near-death experience scientists, both in Europe and America, say that these experiences are simply neurological artifacts. They argue that since taking LSD and other drugs can simulate such experiences (even an endorphin rush during a marathon competition can do it), the sensations reported as near-death experiences are simply part of the brain's innate programming. They suggest that, when someone undergoes the process of dying, brain cells start to break down; the abundance of brain cells in the visual cortex explains why near-death experiences include seeing lights or tunnels of darkness.

Whatever this phenomenon is, people always describe near-death experiences as stimulating a profound transformation. Survivors of near-death experiences connect with their lives differently, they're more appreciative of the things around them, and they desire a deeper spiritual development.

When we die, we ought to have something to say about the way we go, if possible. Do we go with or without tubes and machinery keeping us alive? Do we get electric shock or open-heart massage? We ought to be saying it louder, too, because sometimes it's hard for people to hear, especially people who love us and people who are responsible for our medical care. The Journal of the American Medical Association, reporting on a two-year controlled study of 5,000 patients with life-threatening diagnoses, found that half the doctors didn't know whether their patients wanted to be resuscitated.[8] We need to be talking more clearly to each other, as Carl remembers:

I remember with sadness that when the riddle-maker's time came, I was not ready for him to go and I didn't listen to him. Shortly before his death, Soloho asked me a final riddle. "What happens to the light after it becomes dark?"

I responded, without much hesitation, that since the earth is spinning, and it rotates around the sun, we sometimes face the sun's light and sometimes we face away from it. Darkness is when we are facing away from the sun. He laughed, and for one of the very few times, answered the riddle. He said, "The darkness becomes its own light."

When he came into the hospital, I thought I could set in motion the machinery that would master his life's natural processes. Of course, I couldn't, and he knew that the timing of his final breath would be determined between him and the Creator. My beating on his chest only showed my inability to see his light.

People are becoming disquieted by the cost and the cold technological arrogance of modern medical care. Our fear is that we're going to be kept alive in ways that will destroy our sense of ourselves and burden our loved ones, both financially and emotionally. Lots of people are arguing that doctors should be allowed to end the lives of terminally ill patients in spite of the difficulty in deciding who is terminally ill. What about those patients who are senile and unable to appreciate the consequences, or those families who can't agree? This is not to suggest that there are cases where the termination of life might be merciful. Many doctors have helped people die and will continue to do so. But to legally legitimize this option fundamentally changes the nature of the healing relationship. It can become one that actually encourages self-destruction if your doctor starts thinking you're ready to go, but you are not so sure. You'll pick up those messages, and this is antithetical to the promotion of healing.

You'll also risk losing an opportunity for a unique stage of growth and completion for you and for your family.

A fear that most people have is that of unrelievable pain. In most cases, pain can be effectively controlled using simple techniques, but doctors often don't have the time to listen to their patients, educate them, and support them. Many people are afraid of losing control over their lives and see suicide as the only way to reassert control. The use of ceremonies can be a potent method to reassert control in such situations. A hospice founder who began his service as a home-care volunteer told Howard of this ceremony he instinctively created while visiting a dying patient in her home:

We need to create new ceremonies for the death transition. The hospice movement has been a step in that direction. Hospice care integrates physical, emotional, mental, and spiritual aspects into each patient's care plan.

Grace was a 56-year-old woman with terminal breast cancer. She told me that she knew she was no longer responsive to treatment and just wanted to be with her family and stop her chemotherapy. I knew the family pretty well, and encouraged them to keep her home if they could; I would continue to make home visits. Since I was a pastor and they were atheists, we had always agreed not to talk about religion.

After her discharge, I met with Grace regularly. She talked with me about dying because her grown children had difficulty in listening directly to her thoughts on the subject. She wished she could at least tell her children some things she remembered about her life and hoped they, too, might remember. I knew that her children were all musicians, so I asked them one evening if they would bring their instruments the next time I came. Perhaps they could play for their mother.

The children welcomed the opportunity. The next time I came, they performed a medley of their mother's favorites. The music stretched from a few minutes to an hour. Every week thereafter, for the month before Grace died, they played an informal concert. I brought along some poetry and read it as accompaniment; a friend asked to come and tell a story; slowly the audience grew. Pastor, friends, relatives, each bringing a reading, poem, song, or story. Smiling in her last days, Grace said she wanted us to remember her like this, with such love.

At her funeral service, before the coffin was lowered, her children brought out their instruments and played, I read, her friends told stories. We all thought we saw her smile.

This is Timothy Leary's ceremony for dying, as reported in the *New York Times* on Sunday, November 26, 1995:

Timothy Leary is dying, and he is delighted to talk about it. A sensualist to the end, he is charting his last few minutes on earth, or at least the last few that anyone can be certain of, making sure that the nation's death industry will not spoil this, the experience of a lifetime.

"It's called designer dying," he explained cheerfully into the speakerphone at his house in Beverly Hills the other day. "It's a hip, chic, vogue thing to do. It's the most elegant thing you can do. Even if you've lived your life like a complete slob, you can die with terrific style."

In Tim's very public life, first there was drugs, then Eastern mysticism, media personality, fugitive, stand-up comic and, most recently, cybernetics. And this latest enthusiasm has understandably *absorbed Tim completely. He learned in January that he had inoperable prostate cancer, whereupon he called his old Harvard colleague Ram Dass, among others, to share "the wonderful news" and began the "directed dying" that he had been writing about for 20 years.*

Tim said, "I'm looking forward to the most fascinating experience in life, which is dying. You've got to approach your dying the way you live your life—with curiosity, with hope, with fascination, with courage and with the help of your friends. Let us have no more pious, wimpy talk about death. The time has come to talk cheerfully and joke sassily about personal responsibility for managing the dying process."

Tim is setting up his own event at home, in his bed, with particular attention to that sliver of time between life and death, or near-death and death. "When your heart stops beating, there's a period of 3 to 15 minutes while your brain is still alive," he said. "It's that period that's never really been explored. Everybody has the same story of the near-death experience—my entire life flashed in front of me, the white light and all that—but no one really knows it."

Tim moved life-sustaining equipment into his bedroom, which he called "the de-animation room." He devised a "quality of life index" which, when it got too low, his executors were ordered to pull the plug and release him from his pain. "I can't wait for the moment when I'll have the experience of being in my brain without my body being around," he said. "I'm working on ways of sending signals, my eyebrows moving, that sort of thing."

In April of 1996, Tim developed an Internet web site which actively shared his dying with others. He told us how he was dealing with cancer. His daily diet consisted of 44 cigarettes, three cups of coffee, two glasses of wine, one beer, one marijuana joint, two morphine pills, 12 balloons of nitrous oxide, ketamine, and three "Leary biscuits"—a cheese-soaked marijuana bud on a cracker. Tim Leary was dying as he lived, manifesting his usual New Age philosophy and hilarity.

His friend the author Ken Kesey told him, "Tim, this is our best act so far," and Leary responded, "Yeah, but what do I do for an encore?"

On May 31, 1996, Tim died in Los Angeles. The foremost prophet of psychedelics, dead at seventy-five from prostate cancer. He made funeral arrangements by booking passage for his remains on the "Founders Flight" of a company that carries ashes into space on a commercial satellite. The ashes will eventually plunge in flames into the earth's atmosphere, and Tim will again be scattered among us.

Among the tribes of the Plains, warriors experiencing their final moments sing a death song, the last eloquent expression of one who grasps the fact of his own death. In the face of death, these songs, often spontaneously composed, are chanted with the dying warrior's last breath.

The odor of death
I discern the odor of death
In front of my body
(Dakota)

Among the natives of Hawaii, the elders say that this is the time one receives the Blessing of the Night Rainbow.

There is one night rainbow, the ring that circles the moon, which is a sign of coming weather. There is another night rainbow, much more rarely seen, called Na Po Mokole, "the spirit rainbow." Seen by only a few, it is the rainbow that holds the spirits of all of the ancestors. All of those relatives who have gone out of this flesh come back, and the dying person sees them in the night sky. The spirit family comes back to give the viewer knowledge and strength. Sometimes they can even rekindle one's light when it is weak. The gift of the night rainbow, they say, is the greatest blessing because it kindles the light of unity.

We want our deaths to mean something. These last days can bring heightened awareness, contentment and connectedness. This transition can be as beautiful and profound as the miracle of birth. That's what dying with dignity is about.

Create your own ceremonies for life and for death. The gift of ritual makes your transitions meaningful. In the next section, we will explore how to create personal ceremonies for health.

III

Creating Personal Ceremonies for Health

"It has always been the prime function of
mythology and rite
to supply the symbols
that move the human spirit forward."

—Joseph Campbell

CRAFTING YOUR OWN CEREMONIES

I N THE INTRODUCTION, we described the importance of ceremony in the telling and retelling of one's story and in enhancing connections with other people. We then gave you some examples of how ceremonies can be used during the seasons of our lives. Now we'll show you specifics on how you can create your own ceremonies to help you deal with the transitions in your life.

You don't have to be a medicine person or someone with religious training to be able to craft a ceremony. You can take an existing personal, medical, family, or religious ceremony and modify it to meet the needs of the occasion. At other times you may need to start from scratch, letting your imagination and intuition guide you. Fragments of various ceremonial processes can also be combined for the desired purpose. For example, Howard and Sharona had to be creative:

When we decided to hold a ceremony to help us begin to relate to Arielle's blindness, we visited our rabbi and asked him what the Jewish ceremony for such an occasion was. Fortunately for us, he was very open-minded and replied that there was no "off the shelf" ceremony for such a thing. "That won't stop us," he replied. "We can use some teachings from the Talmud and perhaps include Kaddish (an ancient Jewish prayer of mourning) at the end. Maybe a cedar cleansing ceremony to start." We asked about a Talking Circle, and the rabbi said, "I'm sure we can get it to all fit together."

Putting together a ceremony can be a real challenge. Where do we start? How do we make all the connections for the ceremony? What will we actually do, how will we tell the story, who will run it?

There are four general steps, or building blocks, of a ceremony. These ceremonial components are the frame on which the story will be draped. By following these steps, you can create a ceremony that will add meaning to the experience you share with other participants.

CEREMONIAL BUILDING BLOCKS

The basic steps that lead toward a functional ceremony are identifying the purpose; selecting the community and the facilitator; preparation; and the process of performing the ceremony and the closing. Although ceremonies can be effective when one or more of these components are not fully included, in general eliminating one or more of these steps weakens the effectiveness of the occasion. The first four chapters of this section will explore each of these steps in detail.

Identifying the Purpose

THINK BACK TO a time when you were helped by a ceremony or took part in planning one—a baby shower, a memorial service, a celebration of your job promotion. How could you have woven more meaningful threads into the fabric of the event? At 13, could you have said that what you really wanted for your Bar Mitzvah gift was to go away for a week with your grandfather and uncles and learn how to fly fish and do whatever it is they do when they fish. That sharing of time and experience could have been woven into the framework of the Bar Mitzvah experience.

Look at the important events that have had a big impact in your life—disease, infertility, having children, menopause, and assorted traumas. Could you have dealt with these changes better at the time if there had been ceremonies and all the important people in your life gathered to mark the event with you? Imagine if you could have shared your hopes, fears, and dreams with them more openly.

Ceremonies are ways of telling stories—even painful ones. Ceremonies create times of blessing. Ceremonies provide a structure for getting in touch with our hearts. Ceremonies help us see old certainties in a new way, and something good always happens.

For a ceremony to be most effective, it must have a clear purpose. As you plan your ceremony, think about defining its purpose in terms of what you need and how you hope to grow. For example, we "celebrate" birthdays, but what does that mean? Would it be more meaningful to observe an era with a ceremony to mark the end of one chapter in life and the beginning of something new and promising?

Define your ceremony's purpose specifically, with help from the facilitator and the community (which we'll talk more about later). There are ceremonies of thanksgiving, celebration, blessing, forgiveness, letting go, and affirming in every culture of the world. It is possible for a ceremony to have several purposes, but you should strive to identify "hidden agendas" that might conflict with the main purpose for the ceremony. Remember, every ceremony is created to help participants feel more connected to each other and the story.

The first step in clarifying the purpose of a ceremony is to reflect on how you want to change. What old stories are you clinging to, and how could you rewrite them in a new and better way? Many of the ceremonies described in Section I were designed for this purpose. Howard and Sharona started the design of a special wedding-renewal ceremony by clarifying their purposes:

When we began composing our wedding-renewal ceremony for our fourteenth year of marriage, we felt that there were several purposes. First, we wanted to celebrate our marriage and the simple fact that we had made it this far together. Second, we realized that we had changed as individuals and as a couple over the years and that it was time to let go of some things, such as the making and rearing of babies. Finally, we realized it was time to begin writing a new chapter in our marriage story, one in which we were free to embrace new aspects of the relationship, such as doing some projects as a couple so that we could expand this part of our relationship as our kids got older.

Get clear on the purpose of the ceremony because you will have to describe it, in a couple of sentences, to the other participants. What is it that you wish to happen? That's the purpose of the ceremony. By stating the purpose clearly, you help assure that everybody comes together with the same goal. Howard and Sharona's experience demonstrates how important it is for everyone participating to have clarity about the purpose of the ceremony:

When we were preparing Arielle's ceremony, we began by talking about whom to invite. We agreed that we would like to include one of the staff members from the Foundation for Blind Children, a local agency that had provided support to our family. Upon receiving our invitation, the staff member declined to join us. At first she was evasive about why, but finally she said that she did not want to participate in a ceremony with the goal of restoring Arielle's sight. She carefully explained that she could not lend support to that purpose because Arielle was blind.

Surprised, we explained that that wasn't our purpose at all. It was to let go of our old stories of fear and loss surrounding Arielle's blindness. We wanted to create and share a new story centered around the potential for unexpected gains. Our purpose was to rewrite our stories about Arielle, not hers. Once the staff member understood this, she lent her enthusiastic support and contributed greatly to the event.

Once you have clarified your purpose, you can begin thinking about how you are going to tell this story. In doing so, it may be helpful to look more deeply into the old stories you've already been told. Sometimes it works better to look ahead and write a new chapter in your life story.

Identifying the Community and
the Facilitator

I N HIS BOOK *Black Elk Speaks*,[1] the legendary Oglala medicine man Black Elk says, "A [person] who has a vision is
not able to use the power of it until after he has performed
the vision on earth for the people to see." Once you know
what story (vision) you want to express, you need to identify
both the community and the facilitator who can help you
tell your story in a ceremony.

The facilitator provides the structural threads that keep
attention focused on the ceremony's purpose. At the same
time, the facilitator must allow the event to happen by itself
and not get in the way. You may be the facilitator, or it
could be a priest, a doctor, or even a friend. What's most
important is that it be somebody you trust and who knows
something about performing this ceremony.

Many ceremonies will be initiated by a sponsor. This
person identifies the need for a ceremony and gets things
going to make it happen. The facilitator may be the person
sponsoring the ceremony, or someone recruited because of
his or her expertise in performing such ceremonies. In the
movie business, for example, the "sponsor" is the producer
and the "facilitator" is the director of the film. The facilitator
role can be shared, but this requires careful planning. This
role differs from the usual role of "doctor" in that the facilitator not only strives to "fix" the problem addressed by the
ceremony, but also works to mobilize inner and outer re-

sources. The facilitator imbues meaning into the experience while at the same time being part of the experience.

Facilitators are equally comfortable with trance states, when nothing is happening, as well as with silence and full participation. Their own well-being is enhanced by their participation. Many ceremonial facilitators will train for this role by working as a helper to an experienced facilitator over a period of years. Some people are great facilitators just because of who they are and the life experiences they have had. A first-time facilitator can often do a fine job, particularly if he or she comes to the task with a pure heart and a prepared mind.

Choose the participants in the ceremony with the idea of creating a community. Invite people with whom you want to be on this journey. Get a commitment from each participant to stay at the ceremony from start to finish. Your community may include people at the ceremony and those not physically present. You can include people from the past (ancestors or historical figures), present (friends and relatives who are unable to attend), or future (yet unborn relatives) by mentioning them, through a picture or using other symbols, as Howard did:

When I started cooking the festive meal, it felt like a real ceremony to me. As I was sorting through all of the food, starting water boiling in the pots and cleaning the chicken, I flashed on my grandmothers. As a child, I had watched them cook these foods in just the same way for so many years. It was comforting to be in my own kitchen now, honoring them as I cooked. I decided to take a break from the preparations and went to my old picture album to find pictures of my grandmothers. I brought these pictures back to the kitchen and put them up all around me. We had enjoyed each other's company so many special times over the years in this cooking ceremony. It felt really good to have them watching over me again!

Often just deciding who should attend is itself therapeutic and revealing, as it was for Howard and Sharona:

We had a hard time figuring out where to start on the design of our wedding-renewal ceremony until we focused on the guest list. As we discussed who should (and shouldn't) be invited, we talked about the shared values we wished to express. As we became clearer about who should be there, the purpose and process of the ceremony began to take form.

Reconnecting to community begins when you extend the invitations. Knowing who will be there will help you make preparations.

Preparation

PREPARATION FOR A ceremony is a major determinant of its eventual success. The facilitator and the community share responsibility in preparing the space, the materials, and the process. A ceremony is a time for participants to look within themselves and confront why they are here and what they hope to give and get. A skilled facilitator can follow these threads, planning and preparing the objects and processes to be used in the ceremony.

The facilitator may assign one or more of the participants to do certain tasks before the ceremony is held, as the following story reveals:

It was the first real family vacation we ever took. The kids were just old enough to enjoy traveling in the "house on wheels," an old R.V. we had rented for the trip. We drove north toward Ganado, where we planned to visit two old friends who were working there and were to be married in a traditional Navajo wedding ceremony. We arrived a day or two before the wedding, hoping to explore the surrounding area. When we arrived, we found several families whose members were busy making preparations for the wedding. Some were cooking, some were preparing the space where the wedding would occur, and others were carefully bringing together cornmeal, special baskets, and other items that would be used in the ceremony. I stood outside for several hours cutting vegetables and visiting with the others who had come to attend and help prepare the wedding. It was a wonderful and relaxed way to get to know many of our fellow wedding guests.

As we took our places in the hogan on the day of the wedding, I looked around the circle of faces and felt deeply connected to everyone there. Snapshots of a hundred moments floated past my conscious awareness, forming a collage of emotions and recollections. As the ceremony progressed, the objects that had been so carefully prepared were used, each in its particular way and in its unique place in the ceremony.

Among Native Americans, there is a formal contracting process between the facilitator and the individual sponsoring a ceremony. Sharing the gift of tobacco, they roll a smoke and discuss the purpose of the ceremony.

The preparation phase is actually part of the ceremonial process, especially the developing of connections among participants. A wise facilitator will orchestrate task assignments to bring people together before the ceremony. When properly done, the preparation phase for a ceremony brings joy, comfort, and healing.

SELECTING THE LOCATION

Ceremonies can be performed in tipis or hospital rooms, in caves or cathedrals, in the woods or at the mall, in privacy or at dinner parties. Pick a place that will support the purpose of your ceremony. Find a favorite spot where you won't be interrupted and think about how to work within that space.

GATHERING THE MATERIALS

Materials are gathered and carefully prepared, usually under the supervision of the facilitator. These materials are subsequently used as powerful symbols during the ceremony, particularly those that required a great deal of preparation or that hold special symbolic significance.

Among the materials to be prepared are "sacraments," which are items that affect the senses: hearing (music or drumming), seeing (candle or fire), touching (oils, clothes made of certain fabrics), tasting (ceremonial foods, wine), or smelling (tobacco, cedar, and sage are often used in Native American ceremonies).

Ceremonial objects are items that are used *only* in a ceremonial context (books, antlers, drums, rattles, feathers). Use some that reflect your cultural heritage or that help you focus on the purpose of your ceremony. You probably already have some objects you could include. They may be foods, photographs, a special stone, a Christmas tree ornament that's been handed down for generations, or a piece of clothing. You can also create ceremonial objects, like one of Howard's colleagues did:

The baby had been born with a hypoplastic (underdeveloped) lung on the right side and was to undergo a difficult and dangerous surgery to correct it. I offered to facilitate a preoperative ceremony to help members of the family deal with their feelings about this new child and the upcoming surgery.

We used a black balloon to symbolize the malfunctioning lung, and each participant blew some air into it, talking about the negative emotions they wished to release. In similar fashion, we filled a white balloon with our breath containing our hopes and dreams for this baby. At the end of the ceremony, we went outside and released the air in the black balloon. It looked ridiculous flying around until the air was all gone. The white balloon was tied at the neck and given to the baby's mother, who later placed it by the infant's bedside. The hospital staff, the family and I all understood the greater significance of that simple white balloon.

Sometimes special objects come from surprising places. They may be ordinary items that take on special significance after a birth, death, illness, or other significant event, as in this story of Howard's about his grandfather:

When my grandfather came to our house on Mother's Day, I never suspected it would be the last time I would see him. Four days later he was dead. His health had long been declining, but the suddenness of his death took us all by surprise.

He was the family patriarch, the elder who imparted wisdom, the one to whom everyone listened. This is how I remember him—presiding at the head of the Passover Seder table, all my cousins at one end creating havoc and Grandpa controlling the assembly by picking us off one by one to do the reading. He called us "The Cousins" like it was some sort of club.

We hadn't all been together in more than twenty years. When

we buried my grandfather, though, "The Cousins" left their jobs and families, and everybody showed up at the funeral.

After the burial service we went to my parents' home for the seven-day ritual of mourning. We sat there feeling sad and at the same time strangely hesitant to speak. I invited my cousins to my house the next night. That invitation grew into a dinner just like the big family gatherings we'd had in the old days. We got Chinese takeout food, someone brought wine, another brought dessert, and somebody brought cigars. (My grandfather's favorite thing to do after good food and drink was to smoke a cigar.) When I think of him, I always remember that smell. After dinner, we lit the cigars and got into Grandpa stories. I had some old home movies transcribed onto videotape, so I pulled those out, too. We laughed a lot.

With a sudden inspiration, I jumped up to get some inexpensive shot glasses my mother had found at Grandpa's place. They were the wine glasses we kids used at the Passover Seder, and I told her I wanted to hold onto them.

As soon as I brought the glasses down, everybody recognized them as Grandpa's Passover glasses. "Let's each take one," I said. We decided to use the glasses in future Seders at our homes to represent the Cup of Elijah, the prophet who, legend has it, would herald the Messianic Age.

My grandfather's shot glass has become Elijah's cup. Every Sabbath when I put this little glass on the table, I feel his spirit there with us.

Ceremonial dress may be simple or extensive, depending on the needs of the occasion. Some people may wish to create a piece of clothing for the ceremony, or wear special hats, jewelry, or costumes. Sometimes, the simplest things can become powerful pieces of ceremonial costumes, as Carl describes in this letter to his daughter:

"*Winter '93*

"*My darling daughter,*

"*I'm sitting here in my library looking at these old slippers that last night you half-jokingly said you'd like to keep. I knew they were old but it was only when you called my attention to how scuzzy they appeared that I really looked at them. Usually I'm looking down at these slippers and see only the tops, which look pretty good. Now I'm holding them in my hands, soles facing up, and I'm amazed to see the gaping holes. Bigger holes on the right one remind me of my weak left side. A leftover from the years of back pain and multiple surgeries. I hope I've learned that lesson well, not to ignore my pain until the damage becomes irreversible. Thinking of this reminds me of how you tell me to lighten up in my schedule, maybe take an afternoon nap, and of how much I enjoy working with you. I need to look at this hole in my sole, so I don't get locked into seeing things from only one perspective. Even now I forget to look again, at the things I think I know. I want to give you these old slippers, and thanks for the new ones you sent.*"

My daughter, Lisa, keeps them in a deodorized shoebox along with this letter.

Anything can become a ceremonial object. Franz Kafka told this wonderful story about meeting a little girl in the park one day. The girl was weeping pitifully, because she had somehow lost the doll that she had brought with her. After she spoke with him, it became clear to Kafka that the doll was not going to be found, so he took a piece of paper out of his pocket and said to the little girl that before the doll left, she had left this note for him to read to her: "I can't stand that little room any more. I want to get outside and see what the world is all about. I'll keep in touch with you. I'll send messages and some day, I might even come back. Oh, I may look a little different, but that's because I will have changed some."

The little girl stopped crying. Periodically, Kafka would meet her on his walks in the park, and he'd always read a note to her from her lost friend. Kafka was dying from tuberculosis. He was a young man, and he knew his days were numbered. At a time when his breathing was becoming more labored, he met her once more. This time he brought along another doll.

The little girl asked him what it was and Kafka said, "I think she has changed a little bit, hasn't she?" The girl said, "Is that Brigitta?" Kafka nodded and said, "She came with this note." "Read it, read it to me," the girl pleaded. "I've come home to live with you again. Outside was nice, but coming home is nicer." Then he gave her the doll with the note clenched in its hand. She never saw Kafka again, but the doll became her most precious friend. When she was old enough to read the handwritten note in her doll's hand, she saw that it read, "Everything you love will go away and come back to love you another way."

Suppose Kafka had been a busy man, just exercising briskly in the park. He might have commiserated with her briefly; at best he might have offered to replace the doll with another. Had he done that, it would likely have been rejected because it would have been a substitute when what the little girl really wanted was her best friend. Instead, Kafka told her a story, a story that filled the doll with life and the girl with hope. He created a myth that this girl understood in a deep and intimate way.

We need more storytellers on park benches, in the woods, in front of fireplaces. Stories transform the ordinary events in our lives into lessons, and ordinary objects into links with the extraordinary. Stories that come with a ceremony and/or special objects connect us even more passionately with the loving message, and that's always healing.

Process: Performing the Ceremony

PERFORMING A CEREMONY is more than simply assembling the component parts and saying "Ready, set, go!" Crafting a ceremony requires time, careful attention to detail, and, in most cases, a bit of artistic flair and intuition. One paradox about ceremonies, which is also one of the things that makes these gatherings so powerful, is that they require both careful preparation and openness to spontaneity. Several distinct segments are generally included in a ceremony, and you'll need to be prepared to follow a time-proven sequence of events. But all of your planning is intended to set the stage for people to discover and express their own truths, and for spirit to deliver unexpected blessings.

Each ceremony should have a formal opening that announces, unambiguously, to those assembled, that the ceremony has begun. It's sort of like starting the baseball season by having a celebrity throw out the first ball, or breaking a bottle of champagne on the bow of a ship. During your opening, you need to transform your meeting place into ceremonial "sacred" space that invites special things to happen. You can transform the space by chanting and singing, lighting candles or incense, or saying an invocational prayer. You can use dance, bells, or bugles. When you create sacred space, everyone feels that something special is going to happen here. Carl does when working with his patients:

Before I speak with a patient, I light an oil lamp. Then I ignite some dry sage. This is how I create my office space. I am surrounded by pictures, feathers, kachinas, and ceremonial objects. In winter, wood burns in the fireplace. Patients sometimes ask what I'm doing. I tell them this is a way I dust off the ordinary clingings of the outside world and shelve whatever else is happening in my life so that I can focus on what's happening here between us. This smoke and fragrance give color and substance to our words so that we can hear and understand them in a different way. Something special is going to happen here if we pay attention.

The oil lamp is a reminder of our inner light that sometimes gets covered by lampshades of fear, doubt, and shame until we no longer can see our spirit.

After the opening, the sponsor or facilitator tells the purpose of the ceremony or what are we all doing here. In telling the purpose, you may use pieces of your existing religious practice, ceremonial objects, sacraments, special costumes, or liturgy. One process that works well and is easily adapted to many purposes is the Native American Talking Circle.

The heart of the ceremony is the sequence of activities performed. This process may follow a prescribed blueprint as in some traditional religious ceremonies, or it may be assembled in a creative fashion during the preparation phase. It will usually include sharing of the story through the use of metaphor, symbols, trance, and ceremonial language.

The ceremony should be designed to encourage sharing between participants. They can express themselves through speaking, writing, dancing, movement, or singing. The more you get in touch with symbols and metaphors, the more potent the ceremony becomes. The symbols become the vehicles through which you can express feelings that may not be easy to verbalize.

For example, a father gives his son a prayer shawl that has been passed from father to son for generations and tells him on his Bar Mitzvah, "This connects you to the history of our family and people. One day, God willing, I hope you will give it to your son."

When a ceremony is carefully conducted, it is common for both the facilitator and the participants to experience trance states, which are simply altered levels of awareness. This is not some magical moment that happens to people every day. For example, sometimes time seems to be crawling because you are in a boring lecture, or it can go quickly when you are engaged in intense conversation. Time distortion is an ordinary trance state; so is daydreaming, or concentrating on something so intently that you become unaware of sounds and sights around you.

In a state of trance, you really focus on something. In ceremonies, several elements foster this state. The rhythmic beat of a drum can induce measurable brain wave changes. A fire, sacraments, and language can also promote a trance state. A special language known to the participants is very powerful. The Latin of high mass or sweat lodge songs in Navajo remind you in a powerful way that something special is going on. Howard says:

When we were in Jerusalem, I loved the sound of the prayers being called out from the mosques. Even though I did not fully understand the language, the rhythm and cadence had a special effect. And know-

ing that thousands of worshippers were stopping their activities to bow down in worship of Allah made it a powerful experience indeed!

Finally, each ceremony should have a formal closure that announces unambiguously that the ceremony has ended. This can be done with a special song, blowing out a candle, or a group hug. You just need to find a way to make it clear to everybody when it is time to end the ceremonial circle.

It's not unusual to get a little uneasy before your ceremony, to experience some doubts and fears as the time draws near. Fritz Perls, a well-known psychologist, referred to this feeling of anxiety as "excitement with blocked breathing." Just as in childbirth, breathing is the key to focus and success. As the ceremony begins, it may be helpful to acknowledge this excitement and invite the participants to join you for a few deep cleansing breaths. Howard recalls these feelings:

I still remember the sense of tension as we began the ceremony. I looked around the circle and felt the impact of the presence of these friends and family members. I went from one to the next, smudging each with cleansing cedar smoke as I welcomed and introduced them. It felt good to do this, but my conscious mind worried about being labeled as strange. As I came face to face with my father, then my grandfather, I thought they surely must have thought I had flipped out completely! It was not until the middle of the ceremony that I had the courage to look around the circle again. Much to my surprise, it was obvious that each person was profoundly connected to the proceedings and to each other. Many had tears in their eyes. I realized that I was only a small part of the process and that I could simply let go of my worries and fears. I didn't have to "make it happen"—it was happening on its own.

If your preparation has been thorough, the rest is easy. Let go of the reins once you have moved into the ceremonial space, trusting that your preparations, the energy of the participants, and the healing forces intrinsic to each of us will guide you through.

The Talking Circle

THE TALKING CIRCLE is a simple yet powerful Native American tradition that we have found useful in various settings. A Talking Circle is based on the expectation that everyone participating has something to say and something to learn. This format can create a therapeutic group.

The facilitator traditionally opens a Talking Circle ceremony by burning sage and using an eagle feather to "smudge" the participants, explaining that this is done to wave off whatever clings to us from the outside world, so that we can all be here in this special place. The facilitator may sing a song, offer a prayer, and then express his or her own thoughts about the purpose of the ceremony. You can also open a Talking Circle by lighting a candle or creating sacred space in some other similar way. After speaking, the facilitator passes the eagle feather (or some other object that has special meaning to the group members) to the person sitting beside him or her. That person speaks, then passes the feather to the next person, and so on around the circle.

The ground rules for a Talking Circle are:

- Only one person speaks at a time.
- Each person may speak for as long as he or she wishes, or not at all.
- There is no cross-talk; each person gets one opportunity to speak and only speaks at that time.

- The information shared in the circle can be held in confidence by all participants if they so choose.

Here's an example of an effective use of the Talking Circle that Howard experienced:

When the Foundation for Blind Children asked my wife and me to run a workshop on ceremonies for its Parent and Family Retreat, we wondered how we could ever do so with such a diverse group. After lots of reflection and discussion, we decided to follow a Talking Circle format with a candle as the ceremonial object. The candle would speak powerfully to the participants, who were all parents of visually impaired children.

We knew that several of the parents had not yet accepted their children's disability or had not been able to talk about it. The foundation staff made sure that several experienced counselors would be present to provide support for anybody who needed it after the ceremony. We also trained several staff members to act as facilitators for the four groups of participants.

On the evening of the ceremony, we asked the group's permission to do an experiential exercise. We gave everyone a chance to leave if they were uncomfortable, but nobody did. We reviewed the ground rules for the Talking Circle and asked participants to form four groups of about twelve people each. Then we asked each group to respond to this question: "Describe one negative and one positive aspect of being the parent of a visually impaired child." With some flourish, we lit four candles and gave one to each facilitator.

We moved from group to group to help as needed. Some of the parents answered quickly, and others held the candle for a long time before they could speak. Many were deeply moved, having never shared their innermost feelings with such an understanding, supportive, and safe group. Several of the parents who had been silent about their feelings opened up, their tears reflecting the powerful emotions the ceremony had evoked. As the circles closed, the counselors gently approached those individuals and asked if they might want to talk privately. All said yes, and many stayed for hours working with the counselors.

Here's another example of a Talking Circle that Carl ran in which some unexpected elements led to a great healing:

I'd been invited by the Milton Erickson Institute in Köln, Germany, to deliver a seminar there. For a long time I delayed accepting because I've long been filled with bad feelings about Germans. I am a child of Holocaust survivors, and that fact has had a profound influence on every aspect of my life. German was my mother tongue, but I spoke it only to members of my family, never to Germans. I have carried with me, thinly veiled beneath my civility, a sense that all Germans share some culpability for the Nazi era.

I knew I could not go to Germany to teach while I felt this way. Things were bound to come up that I was not prepared to hear. I knew most of the participants would be younger than I, but could I shelve my old judgmentalism and not wonder what role their parents had played during World War II?

I couldn't hold on to that much anger for so many years without it affecting my ability to heal myself and to touch others in healing ways. So I decided to go to Germany. I conducted the seminar on the 50th anniversary of the liberation of Auschwitz. It was, for me, an announcement of my own liberation.

On the first day of the Milton Erickson Institute meeting in

Cologne, I delivered a lecture on trance induction and how to create healing stories to a group of physicians, psychologists, social workers and other care providers. On the second day, I announced that the previous lecture would be translated into a ceremony. I described the Native American Talking Circle as a place where we could come together and express ourselves without fear or judgment. We would use all of the elements of ceremonies that we had discussed to create a mood to pay attention to what would be said here.

I told the group that the candle flame in the middle of our circle reminded us of the light within each of us, the light of our spirit selves. It is that piece of us that propels us forward during the adversities in our lives. Sometimes our flame becomes dimmed by fear and doubt until the shade gets so dense that no light shines through. I understand the process of psychotherapy as helping people take off their lampshades so that they can remember the light within.

Then I pointed to the abalone shell in which I had placed some sage, given to me by an Indian relative. He had picked it in a special place in the forest that had been shown to him by his father, whose father before had shown it to him. I lit the sage and waved its fragrance over the circle, saying, "Imagine that whatever thoughts and preoccupations keep you from being here in this moment are being washed away." I walked around and waved an eagle feather over each participant. The eagle feather was given to me by a Sundancer; they believe that our words get carried skyward on the wings of eagles to touch the ear of the Creator. "You will hear each others' words, and now we can see them and smell them. Some things will be said here that need to be heard," I said.

When I finished "smudging" everyone, I sat down and spoke in German. I told of my old fears and judgments, and of my difficulty in deciding to come here. I said that my childhood fears mirrored my *father's belief that at any moment everything could be taken from you; you could never be too secure. I spent much of my time writing and speaking about truth and perceptions, I told the circle, and I wanted to be able to walk my talk and reconsider my old stories.*

Nervously, I passed the feather and allowed the circle to happen. I heard that there were indeed people here whose parents had been Nazis or members of the Hitler Youth. But my worst fantasies were not realized. There was also someone whose father was killed as a member of the Resistance movement. In an extraordinary event that took hours, I finally saw the children of other survivors. In that ceremonial setting, a place without judgment, where the expectation was that something good would happen, something did.

By the time the feather came back to me and 28 people had spoken, I knew that I was different. And I knew in my heart, not just in my mind, that there was a difference between Germans and Nazis. As I closed the circle, I held the feather and spoke to my father. I said that his greatest fear—that we would not survive as families and as a people—had not materialized. I was sitting here in the country of his birth as testimony to our survival, and I was here with others who had also survived.

The Talking Circle is a moving way to get all participants involved in the process of the ceremony. Find an object to pass around that will "speak" to the participants, and trust that it and the setting will draw out each individual's truth. Let people express themselves as fully as they need to. Only rarely will you need to intervene if somebody gets "stuck" during the circle. Howard was invited to give a lecture on medical ceremonies at Stanford University:

I was flooded with memories of my time there as a medical student. Inside this temple of science, I listened to stories of patients' suffering and triumph. Several people from the Medical School attended. Each of these people had treated me with kindness and respect during medical school, and I wanted to thank them in a special way.

I arrived early on the day of the lecture and ceremonially set up the conference room. I moved the tables into a large rectangle so that we could all sit around it in a circle, as if we were at the proverbial kitchen table. I lit some cedar and sage and "smudged" the room and said a prayer. I prayed that something good would come as a result of this meeting about to take place.

One by one, people started arriving for the lecture, lunch in hand. I began by lighting a small candle and talking about what I had learned about why ceremonies are important in caring for patients. I presented all of the components of a ceremony while everybody sat munching their lunches. I explained that surgery, psychotherapy, childbirth, medical procedures, rounds, conferences, code arrests, office visits, and even meals like this one can all be important ceremonial events.

As everybody finished lunch, I asked them to relax in their seats and allow their minds to drift. Thoughts might drift by, but they need not dwell on them. With another part of their awareness, I asked them all to picture a reservoir holding water, each picturing it in his or her own way and taking notice of the fullness of the water. Was the reservoir inside each of them empty, or was it overflowing? I suggested each person spend a few moments allowing the reservoir to be filled by rain, incoming streams, friends forming a bucket brigade, or whatever suited them. Each at his own pace and in his own way refilled his reservoir and then returned back to the conference room.

Then I picked up the lit candle and explained the ground rules *for the Talking Circle. I asked each to share whatever he wanted to about their visualization experience when the candle came to him. As the candle began its way around the circle, everybody began to realize that this was more than a lecture. We were joined as a community connected within this ceremonial circle, renewing our ties and our energy.*

When the candle came back to me, I thanked the group for sharing their experiences and for sustaining me during medical school. I blew out the candle, and hugs broke out all around.

The Talking Circle's power is in its simplicity.

Medical Participation

THERE'S A GROWING interest in the use of ceremonies for change and healing.[2,3,4,5] But we have yet to fully incorporate healing ceremonies into medical practice. A recent study of alternative therapies, including ceremonial practices, found that "individuals using such therapies were more likely to have chronic illnesses [than those who did not use such therapies] and 72 percent of the respondents did not inform their medical doctor that they had done so."[6]

CEREMONIES AND MEDICAL TRAINING

It is not surprising that physicians have lost their ceremonial skills, since the use of ceremonies is rarely mentioned explicitly during their training. That lack of mention is surprising, since many of the methods of training are highly ceremonial, including hospital rounds, lecture discussions, and morning reports.

Water is a potent symbol for the connecting life force and is useful in many ceremonies. Here's an example of a medical training ceremony that Howard derived from an ancient water ceremony practiced by the Sufi mystics of Persia:

On July 1 each year, there is a big turnover in hospital medical personnel. That's the day new interns and residents begin their training. When I became an intern, the day was filled with fear and anticipation. I knew what I knew, but I didn't yet know what I didn't know. One day I was a medical student and the next I was suddenly an intern. I knew that sooner or later, I'd face a real life-or-death situation, and I wondered how I would respond.

The first day, the other seven interns and I met in the conference room and were greeted with a brief speech. This was followed by a list of our duty assignments and, finally, our pagers. That was the ceremony of our initiation. Years later, after becoming the Director of the Family Practice residency program, I devised a new welcoming ceremony.

The incoming interns formed a small circle in the middle of the room and the senior residents and faculty formed another circle around them. I sat in the inner circle with the interns and welcomed them to our training family, saying, "We are a family that depends on each other. We will teach you everything we know, and we want you to use it for good. Today you move from student to doctor. You will begin to learn about integrating the art and the science of healing.

"There is a Sufi water ceremony in which each member of the group receives from and gives to the others his hopes and prayers through the sharing of communal water. I'm going to pass these cups around; please take one. Our residency coordinator will fill each of our cups from this communal pitcher. The water is a gift of life. We want to nurture you, to commit our competence to you, and watch you grow. As you look at this water, imagine you are putting into it what you are willing to give to your patients and to this residency, and to each other. Think also about what it is that you need to receive from yourself, from your colleagues, and from us."

Then, one by one, everyone spoke of their enthusiasm, of their caring, of their hopes and fears. As each finished, he emptied his cup back into the pitcher. When the circle was completed, I invited the faculty advisors to once again fill the interns' cups from the water that had been poured from the cups back into the pitcher. Silently, each faculty member did so. As each of them looked into the eager eyes of their advisees, they recognized a part of themselves. In that moment, they connected in a special way with each other.

I told them to drink half of the water in their cups and said, "This is a very important moment in your lives and in the life of this residency. Each of you is about to go through the trials of training in hopes of emerging as a doctor and a healer. We acknowledge this moment and embrace it with you. From this point on we are connected together. We happily accept the gifts that you are willing to offer and commit ourselves to help you in every way we can to learn and grow. Moses Maimonides, a physician who practiced over 800 years ago, meditated on this prayer every day before seeing patients:

You have chosen me to watch over the life and health of your creatures. I am about to apply myself to the duties of my profession. Almighty God, support me in this great work that it may benefit my fellow creatures; without your help, even the least thing will not succeed. Inspire me with love for my occupation and for your creatures. Permit not thirst for profit or ambition for renown to interfere with my profession. These enemies of truth can lead us astray in the great task of attending to the well-being of your creatures. Preserve my physical and spiritual strength that I may cheerfully be of help to rich and poor, good and bad, friend and foe alike. Let me see only the human being in the sufferer.

*   *   *

I invited the other residents and faculty to share whatever words they might want to. Our chief resident said, "I know you are all nervous— I felt the same way. I just want you to know that you will survive this. We are all here to support you on your journey." Several other people spoke movingly from their hearts to the interns.

It was time to close the ceremony. "From this point on, I officially welcome you to our training family and wish you well on your road toward becoming doctors and healers." Each of the interns drank from the water remaining in his cup. Each was connected in a new and special way.

CEREMONIES AND MEDICAL TREATMENT

Sooner or later a serious medical problem will bring you face to face with the core issues—mortality and the meaning of life, among others. Ceremonies can strengthen the physical and emotional healing processes at these times by pulling together the most essential elements you need—the love of the important people in your life, deeply felt prayers and healers who can help you face your fears and worries.

We believe ceremonies work synergistically with medical procedures, not just in parallel with them. If you're facing your own or a loved one's medical crisis, you may be able to include your physician, nurses, or other health-care providers in a healing ceremony. Knowing that the people responsible for your physical recovery are also committed to you spiritually can be a powerful tool for healing. Howard used this tool during a personal illness:

I was very proud of myself after I lost the first five pounds, but after I lost another twenty without really trying, I started to get concerned. As a physician, I knew that cancer could be one reason for this, so I decided to make an appointment with my personal physician, who used to be a student of mine. As the nurse took my blood pressure, I was surprised that it was significantly elevated. My mind started to recognize what my body already knew—something was going on here. When my doctor, Steve, entered the room, he came over and gave me a big hug. I could feel my blood pressure fall ten points just from this wonderful hug. "Tired? Fevers? Any blood in your stool?" He clicked through all the right questions. "We'll have to run some tests to sort this out. Don't worry—we'll get to the bottom of this."

When I was at work later that week, Steve called and explained that my thyroid blood test was quite high. He suggested I see an endocrinologist for further diagnostic testing. A few days later, I was sitting in the endocrinologist's office. Phil was an older man who had been trained as a classical internist. I thought about how pleasant it was to be able to sit clothed and comfortable in his consultation office. He took me to his examining room for a physical exam, then we both walked back to his consultation office. He said, "You'll have to go for a thyroid scan—it's really quite simple—then we'll know better how to treat this."

The night before the thyroid scan, I asked my wife to loosely tie some thread around my wrist. I knew that I would have to be alone and lying still for long periods of time during this procedure, and I wanted this thread to be able to remind me of my ties to family and friends. As she tied the knot, she blessed me and expressed her love and concern for me. Ah, the best medicine there is!

The next day, I walked into the outpatient registration area, where I waited with other patients until I was finally called by the intake person. She asked me about my insurance and then fastened a plastic hospital bracelet on my wrist, right over the threads placed lovingly by my wife the night before. I felt that the thread was my inner self covered by a plastic, computer-generated hospital wristlet— my outer self.

The radiologist explained that the radioactive capsule I was to swallow would collect in my thyroid. That way we could scan the gland and figure out its activity level. He put on some latex rubber gloves, opened a small, lead-lined bottle that looked much like a prescription bottle, placed a capsule on the cover of this bottle, and handed me a glass of water. I reached to pick up the capsule and he said no, he would pop it into my mouth directly from the lid. Great, I thought, too hot to handle but not too hot to swallow!

I then was taken to the scanner, a large machine with a silver metallic cone whose tip was pointed an inch from my neck. The technician told me that I could not swallow or move for several minutes. That turned out to be quite difficult, and during these times I felt the thread around my wrist and remembered my wife, my kids, my friends, and my teachers. In that instant, the doctor had become the patient, and I saw my world in a new way. I looked for something alive in this high-tech room, and my gaze fell on a single potted plant near the window. I decided that I wanted to live. Whatever they found, I wanted to continue to be connected with the important people in my life.

I did not have cancer, but I did have Graves' disease, a condition of the thyroid frequently associated with an overactive thyroid. It's not going to kill me, but it is important to pay attention to it. My "illness" has served to bring into focus what is important in my life, what sustains me. I also felt compassion and kinship with patients, many of whom have faced situations far more formidable than mine.

My physician gave me a prescription for a medication that would slow down the activity in my thyroid gland. It was hard for me to start taking it, so I put it off for the week of Passover. During the seder meal, I tasted the unique flavor of the matzoh and burned my mouth with horseradish. After the meal, I took my first pill for "dessert." As we learn from the Passover story, from adversity comes growth.

Several days later, I conducted a Passover/Easter sweat lodge ceremony at our home. Lots of friends came. My wife's prayers touched my heart as she prayed for me to return to balance, energy, and strength. Others expressed their love and concern for me in ways that touched my heart, and that's when I knew that the healing had occurred. I would continue to take the medication, but it was now only a detail, just another maintenance procedure to keep my body healthy. I had returned from the "Graves'." Transform life's challenges into life-changing experiences that help you find ways to keep connected with the important threads in your life.

Although some doctors have a warm and creative relationship with their patients, many are convinced that they must remain objective or in charge and not become emotionally involved. A doctor who tells jokes or invites you to draw caricatures on his white coat is sharing more than his professional expertise with you. The rare physician may give you talismans—a little cloth friendship bracelet to wear in the Magnetic Resonance Imaging (MRI) machine or a special stone picked up during a walk in the woods. Such simple gestures communicate that your doctor is working with you and trying to help take your mind off your claustrophobia or dread. A simple condolence letter to a deceased patient's family lets them know their doctor is aware that he or she may have lost a patient, but that you've lost a loved one.

The practice of medicine does in fact contain many elements of ceremony, but they're not always geared toward the patient's well-being. Executive sessions of medical staff meetings have a "ceremonial" opening. A special legal "invocation" is read to keep the proceedings confidential. At the end of the meetings, all the written materials (printed on a special blue paper and serially numbered) are carefully passed back to the leader of the group.

Technologically sophisticated medical procedures often involve a highly specialized language, one that has powerful meaning for the physicians but is usually foreign to patients. These ceremonies help the medical staff create a community of support. The operating room contains a lot of ceremonial activity, including special costumes and medication "sacraments" (i.e., anesthetic agents for the patient and coffee for the OR team). Operating rooms are frequently equipped with radios and CD players because doctors are more relaxed and work better when they can hear music they like.[7]

Music also helps alleviate the *patient's* anxiety just before surgery. Choosing the music you'd like to hear before you're anesthetized for surgery gives you some control over this event in which you're entrusting your life to others; it also says that the medical staff cares about your total well-being, not just your malfunctioning organ.[8] Many hospitals now have birthing rooms to encourage family involvement. Women often bring music, incense, and other "sacraments" to be used during their labor.

The medical policy of "informed consent" requires that before doing a medical procedure, the physician must describe to the patient the steps in the procedure and explain the risks and benefits. You must sign a legal form saying that you consent to the procedure. This discussion allows you to be sure you understand what's involved, to ask questions, and to decide whether to have the procedure. This meeting with the doctor also gives you an idea of when and how ceremonial components could be added to your treatment.

For instance, it is reasonable to ask your physician to obtain for you the organs removed during surgery (uterus, gallstones) or the afterbirth so that you can dispose of it ceremonially. Native Americans bury the placenta; the Vietnamese do a blessing ceremony with it.

When you feel emotionally connected to your doctor, and can participate in decisions about your care, you share control of and responsibility for the outcome.

WHAT IF MY DOCTOR WON'T JOIN IN?

Some physicians will enthusiastically join in a ceremony to help promote healing. Others, like Sharona's surgeon in Section I, will respect your choice and not interfere, but also decline to participate. Yet others will ridicule what you're doing. If your doctor doesn't want to join in, you can still craft a ceremony yourself.

Elective surgery presents a wonderful opportunity to re-examine and transform stories about your identity, even without the active participation of the surgical team. You can do this with friends or with guidance from a therapist before surgery. Sometimes a medical treatment that you choose to have represents a turning point in your life, as Howard's wife Sharona explains:

Many issues from my first 40 years were keeping me stuck and anxious. They centered around my fear of being alone and unloved if I was needy, dependent, and imperfect. I worked hard to suppress these fears by careful diligence, some compulsiveness, and a bit of denial. But there was one part of my being that I could not deny—my spine was increasingly curving to a dangerous point, and extensive surgery was necessary to prevent debilitating disability and pain in later years.

Since my early teens, I'd dealt with the disfigurement of scoliosis.

I chose to do this silently and privately. I wore my back brace only at home with my family, so friends never knew of this "apparatus" that was part of my life. Doctors discussed surgery as an option, emphasizing that it would mean a dangerous procedure followed by a year in a body cast and a lengthy stay in bed. The myriad physicians my parents consulted felt this wasn't necessary, since in most cases, scoliosis did not worsen after childhood. However, as I was to learn later, it can progress and cause major disability and early death if left untreated.

As I grew into adulthood, married, and had children, I continued to ignore my physical condition. Dealing with it might result in having to confront my anxieties over dependency and imperfection. In my late 30s, after seeing an older friend who was suffering great pain from her scoliosis, I decided to have some X-rays taken. Timidly, I visited an orthopedic surgeon, hoping for a stable prognosis, only to hear the surgeon strongly recommend an operation for my advancing curvature.

The room seemed to spin as I realized I could not deny my situation any longer. I had to face the old fears and the new ones that would arise if I underwent surgery: possible long-term effects, hospitalization, dependency, stresses on my husband and children, and my greatest fear—loss of love.

Fortunately, my husband and I had been through a lot together, and we had learned the wisdom of thoughtfully dealing with fears and using them as opportunities for growth, lessons, and transformation. Despite tremendous anxiety and the desire to get this episode over as soon as possible, I decided to spend a year preparing for my surgery (there was little medical risk in doing this), using various resources to transform my situation into a positive one. There were many difficult times, but also many precious and sweet ones. . . .

First, I spoke honestly and openly with those closest to me about my fears and concerns. Friends reassured me that they'd be there to help in any way I needed. Once I was confronting my fears, I was eager to find healthy ways to cope with them. One friend, a psychologist and highly skilled hypnotherapist, offered to help me prepare for the surgery through hypnosis. Through his guidance, I learned how to take my conscious and unconscious minds to places of serenity—beside the ocean or to a bubbling brook in the woods. In my mind, I invited loved ones from my present and my past to join me and comfort me in these surroundings. I learned how to enter a more relaxed space (or "trance") when I felt uptight, when I had trouble sleeping, and when I had to go through uncomfortable medical procedures. Instead of spending anxious moments imagining the surgery and possible outcomes, I was able to fantasize about splashing in warm water or basking in the sunlight. This, I see now, was the preparation phase of my transformational ceremony.

I worked with the therapist for over half a year on positive messages for relaxation, surgical preparation, and dealing with post-surgical pain or discomfort. I used my tapes and messages before and after surgery. I could reconnect at any time to my stronger, calmer self who felt in control and was competent and loved.

I dealt with my fears of alienation and potential loss of support by inviting those close to me into my "drama," to be part of my unfolding story. I was warmly reassured of my friends' concern and availability, and people helped in many creative ways. Before the surgery, a number of close friends presented me with small gifts or tokens of healing (music, pictures to meditate on, other items) and reminders of their love. During surgery and recuperation, several prayer groups included me in their prayers, and I am certain that their thoughts contributed to my healing. During rehabilitation at home, many friends and neighbors brought my family nourishing meals and treats.

My surgery—my transformational ceremony—was a medical success. And in the process, I learned of the love and support that surrounds me. My hospital room and home were filled with flowers, plants, and cards. New modes of healing touch comforted me—the hair-washing experience (described in Section I) and soothing post-operative massages. I learned that support can come in many ways if you're open to it and tell others of your need for it.

After the surgery, every moment seemed a miracle. Facing lifelong fears helped me rewrite my life's script and brought me the power of knowing I could deal creatively with whatever challenges were ahead.

Once I was again strong and agile, my husband and I sponsored a sweat lodge ceremony to thank and honor all of those who had played an important role in my healing. I carefully cut up the orthopedic T-shirts I had worn under my brace into small squares. We made ceremonial prayer bundles out of these by filling each square with some tobacco and a prayer, tying them shut, and stringing them together. As I sat in the sweat lodge and looked at all of these bundles hanging from the willow ribs, I was awed by this miracle of transformation.

With a little help from your friends, the courage of the spirit can transform fear into growth.

Closing

WHEN WE BEGAN this venture several years ago, we hoped to share a journey that reflected our experiences as medical doctors who expanded their scientifically based healing repertoire. We laughed and we struggled with each other, because it's not easy for two people to write with one voice. It's hard to give up old preconceptions and come to each other in a new way. We are teachers, students, children, lovers, wives, husbands, etc., and that's the way it always is. We have a tendency to keep seeing the light through old lampshades.

We have moved from mentorship to friends. We have come to each other as we come to the world, listening to stories and telling our own. Our destiny is not transmitted genetically, but rather through our stories. It is through sharing our journeys that we make sense of our life experience.

These are the stories we've learned along our paths. As doctors, we knew the journey to healing is a process, not a recipe. Incorporate those elements that speak to your heart and weave them into your ceremonial life. These are vehicles that can take you on your own journey of discovery.

This is the way the Lubavitcher Rebbe told the story:

During the once-a-year personal consultation the Rebbe counseled one of his Hasidim, Moishele, to pray (daven) with greater vigor and intention. Moishele humbly said, "Show me how, Rebbe. I only know the words." But the Rebbe really didn't want to answer him, because the soul of davenning is not easy to teach. Instead, the Rebbe called in his deputy, and told him to tell Moishele how to daven with passion. But the deputy also demurred and instead called in the head of the yeshiva, who was "the last man on the totem pole." So the head of the yeshiva began to daven the morning service right there on the spot. Together they all prayed until the head of the yeshiva came to a point in the service when he announced, "And now when I get to this part, that's a place for me alone," and he walked off to a corner by himself, pulled his prayer shawl over his head, and prayed. The Lubavitcher Rebbe leaned over to Moishele and said, "That's davenning. It's improvising in the private place."

It doesn't matter how the story is told; we are well-trained doctors of medicine but we are also ambassadors from Jerusalem, Dar es Salaam, Bear Butte, and Mecca. Our consultation rooms are filled with objects, photographs and aromas, all of which are connected to their own stories and ceremonies. They all help us create an atmosphere that promotes a relationship between doctor and patient. It is through relationships that we strengthen our power, and it is through relationships that we sustain ourselves when we are broken.

We came from different walks, but we always managed to get together in ceremonial space. So when we finished the book, we gave this blessing to each other:

"Thank you, Creator of all things, for bringing us together in this way.
Thank you for helping us tell this story in the best way we know.
Bless my brother on his journey."

Ceremony Planning Worksheets

I. PURPOSE

Carefully consider your purpose in creating and performing this ceremony. What is it that you want to accomplish, witness, share, and/or demonstrate?

The purpose of this ceremony is to:

_____

_____

The parts of my "old story" that I want to release are:

_____

_____

_____

_____

_____

The important aspects of my "new story" that I want to tell
are:

_____

_____

_____

_____

_____

_____

_____

_____

_____

_____

_____

_____

Who should facilitate the ceremony, and who needs to be there? The time and place of your ceremony may determine the availability of the facilitator and community. Are there individuals who cannot be physically present whom you want to invite to participate "in spirit"?

Facilitator: _____

List of Participants: _____   _____

_____   _____

_____   _____

_____   _____

_____   _____

_____   _____

_____   _____

III. Preparation

There are several questions to address in order to prepare for a ceremony:

- How should the ceremony be opened and closed?

- Where should it be held, and what needs to be done to properly prepare the space?

- What process is conducive to achieving the desired purpose, and how structured should this process be?

- How should the participants be notified and included in the preparation?

- What types of special objects, dress, or sacraments will be used, and who will gather them and how?

NOTES:

_____

_____

_____

IV. PERFORMING THE CEREMONY

Make a rough script of how the various elements will be performed. Who will do what parts of the ceremony, and how will it flow?

Ceremonial Step	Who will perform?	Materials required
Opening	_____	_____
Process	_____	_____
Closing	_____	_____

A Special Request to Our Readers

We ask that you share your healing journeys with us. If you have found ways to bring ceremony into your life and your healing, please write to us and share your stories:

T.I.P.I. / Ceremonies
3104 East Camelback Road, #614
Phoenix, AZ 85016

Carl Hammerschlag's
Ceremonial Calendar

These are the things I use in my life. There are many other once-in-a-lifetime ceremonies that also occur.

DAILY
— ✺ —

- On awakening I do a half hour of yoga; I breathe and listen to the voice of emptiness. This relaxes me and helps me move from my bed to the workaday world.

- I do a morning-greeting blessing in my back yard. As the sun is coming up over the Camelback Mountains and I see the Praying Monk outlined in gold, I open my arms and start, something like this . . .

  Tunkashila, Grandfather, Ribbono Shel Olam . . . good morning, thank you for all the blessings in my life; to be able to greet you standing on two legs, to be able to walk upon the earth, to be here with my family, my relatives, my friends, my patients. Thank you for my teachers and my students, for all the blessings I have in my life, for the ones that I get and the ones that I give . . .

✺

Then I will pray for relatives if they're sick, for the world during our unnatural cleansings, or whatever happens to be on my mind at the moment.

The word "blessing" is both a verb and a noun, which means it's something you give and something you can receive. Blessings start your day off with a smile.

- I start every day with fruit. I eat lots of vegetables now; no meat, chicken or dairy products. I've been doing this for the last year, and my blood pressure has come down. I say thanks for this blessing.

- Almost every day I swim a mile. The first few years it was boring because I counted the laps. When I decided to swim for 40 minutes instead and stopped counting, it freed my mind to wander. Now I daydream, sometimes even find a solution to a problem.

WEEKLY

- When I see my patients, I first light a candle and burn some sage in a shell that was given to me by my mentor/uncle. I tell my patients why I do this, and then together we separate ourselves from whatever is happening outside our space in the world beyond our doors so that we can refocus on what's happening right here and so that we can speak to and listen to one another in a special way. I begin every psychotherapy session with this trance induction.

• During midweek, when the work seems heavy, I get an hour-and-a-half massage. Before the massage, I light a candle or the fireplace, then I put on some of my favorite CDs (Enya, Kitaro, Pachelbel's Canon in "D" with Ocean Sounds, Carlos Nakai, William Eaton, Andreas Vollenweider, Mannheim Steamroller) and then I lie down for a while to separate my head from my body. With deep muscle massage I disconnect from this world, and it restores my energy.

• On Friday night of every week I celebrate the Sabbath with song and dance and family. Now that I'm older, with grandchildren, I feel the importance of ancestors and teachings. I say thank you for giving me a tribe and an ethical way to walk in this life.

PERIODICALLY

• When I first came to Indian country in 1965, the most important questions people asked were not where I got my degrees or did my training. They wanted to know if I could pray from my heart in my own language. I really didn't know. I knew I could pray in my language, but I never felt like I could talk to God.

Indians invited me into the tipi anyway, and in there, with that awesomely powerful sacrament, I revisited my relationship with God. In the tipi of the Native American Church, I learned how to talk to the Spirit. I developed a relationship with the Spirit above and with the one within. In the tipi was the first time I was able to speak to God without feeling angry. When I was young, I only prayed when I was afraid, which developed into an interestingly hostile-dependent relationship with God. God always reminded me of my weakness, so I railed against God because I didn't like to be reminded of what I know to be true about myself but don't especially like to face. I pray a lot more now.

YEARLY

— ❦ —

- Every year I go on a fishing trip into the White Mountains, to a remote lake on the White Mountain Apache Reservation where I spend four days with my sons-in-law and a close friend I call brother. As soon as we reach the Maricopa County line, we become transformed into our "truckin'" personas.

Jay, the in-your-face attorney, is called The Basic Advocate. Max, the quintessential peddler, is The Junkman; John, the scientist/philosopher, becomes The Cosmic Peg, and I am simply The Mouth.

It takes us 40 minutes to arrive in Globe, Arizona, where we stop for lunch at the El Rey Cafe. It's been run by the same family for 40 years. They serve their handmade tortilla chips drenched in butter. (The only thing missing at the El Rey is a cardiac resuscitation unit in the parking lot.) We dip those invitations to death into their guacamole with the speed of athletes competing in an Olympic event. By the time this tribute to overindulgence is over, we can barely get into the van. We drive to our secret swimming hole at the bottom of Salt River Canyon. Then it's on to Pinetop, where The Cosmic Peg directs our shopping spree. Everyone picks a favorite thing from smoked oysters to Captain Crunch and beers from around the world.

Then we move into the desolation. Fifty rugged miles through exquisite countryside. Snow-capped peaks, elk, bear, beaver, mountain lion, eagles, and osprey. We fish, bathe in the ice-cold water, eat and drink like followers of Pan. This time regenerates me. It always reminds me to appreciate the familiar in new ways. I need to do this to stay alive.

- Every year I go to a Jewish Renewal gathering and get together with other members of my tribe who have found some extraordinary ways to tell the old stories.

Howard Silverman's
Ceremonial Calendar

These are the ceremonies that I do on a regular basis:

- Every day upon wakening, I go out the front door of our home and walk to my workshop, where I carefully put on tallis and tefillin (the ritual bindings of my faith that I drape around my shoulders and strap to my arm and forehead) and get centered. This is a sort of time to check in, to "calibrate" myself to face the rest of the day.

- I always make sure I give each of my daughters a hug and a kiss before dinner.

- Our family has always had dinner together, except under very unusual situations. We spend this time sharing stories from the day, consciously waiting until after dinner to get into any negative stuff. If there are any issues that need to be solved, any member of the family can call a family meeting during dinner (also described in Section II). Usually we discuss the issue at hand and have always been able to reach a solution that everybody can accept. More than anything else, I believe this has taught our children that problems can be solved in a way that enhances relationships.

- Every evening, I sit outside for ten or fifteen minutes and look at the stars. This is a wonderful time for letting go of the day's tensions.

- When I come in from my stargazing time, I share a healthy snack of low-fat pretzels and sliced apples with my wife and daughters.

WEEKLY

- I swim laps three times a week for about a half hour without fail. Afterwards, I try to consciously slow down a bit in preparation for returning home.

- When seeing a patient, I am careful to establish the purpose for the visit while he or she is seated comfortably in a chair. When it is time to perform the physical exam, I ask the patient to move to the exam table. I try to perform some type of exam on every patient, even when it is not medically necessary, because I believe this physical connection has important ceremonial effects.

- Every Friday night, we gather as a family around the kitchen table. My wife lights the Sabbath candles, and my daughters join her in singing the blessings.

I really love to close my eyes and drift away on the sound of their voices joined in blessing and song. Then my eldest daughter or I sing the blessing over the wine followed by a blessing over the food sung by all of us.

• On Saturdays, I relax with my family and do *no* work whatsoever.

PERIODICALLY

• We do sweat lodge ceremonies several times per year, usually connected with Jewish holidays. This ritual requires a lot of heavy physical work to prepare, and I have learned to allow enough time for this work so that it becomes a sort of meditation.

• Whenever I feel my energy level going down, I enjoy spending a day at home preparing chicken soup, as taught to me by my grandmother. Then I eat the soup over the next few days, allowing it to nourish and cleanse my body.

• Once or twice a year I try to get away for a day or two to hike in the desert. I always hike alone. As the years have rolled by, I have found myself covering less territory and spending more of my time in one place. I usually bring a home-wrapped cedar and sage bundle and spend an hour or two after lunch in meditation while this prayer bundle slowly burns, filling the air around me with its fragrant smell.

ANNUALLY

- There are a host of ceremonies connected with the annual cycle of the family practice residency training program in which I work. It really is a lot like farming, with a time to "plant" and to harvest (the new interns arrive in the summer and the senior residents depart). We always have a large banquet to commemorate the departure of our graduating residents, and we invite families as well as alumni.

  When our new interns arrive, I stage a ceremony to welcome them based on the Sufi water ceremony (described in Section III).

- Each year I try to get away to the desert for a day or two before the Jewish New Year. I use this time to get centered, to review my life, and to consider those areas of my life that are in need of reevaluation and repair.

VERY SPECIAL CEREMONIES

- Every seven years, my wife and I perform a wedding-renewal ceremony. These ceremonies have helped us to renew our commitment to each other, to make it more relevant to where we are now.

- Recently, we celebrated the Bat Mitzvah of our oldest daughter. This was really a week filled with powerful and sustaining ceremonies, culminating in her Bat Mitzvah service. Relatives and friends joined us from near and far, and it was wonderful to see everybody reconnecting with each other. As our daughter deftly led all of us in prayer, I began to realize that our daughter was no longer a child. This is one of the purposes of this adolescent transition ritual, and it helped all of us to leave childhood behind.

References

SECTION I—ABOUT CEREMONIES

1. Hammerschlag, Carl A. *The Dancing Healers*. New York: HarperCollins, 1988.

2. Torah Aura Productions. "Learn Torah With . . ." Commentary on Genesis 44:18–47:27. Vol. 1, No. 11, Dec. 10, 1994, page 1.

3. Chopra, Deepak. "Timeless Mind, Ageless Body." *Noetic Sciences Review*, 28:17–21,1993.

4. Jung, Carl Gustav. *Psychological Types*, p. 82. A Revision by R.F.C. Hull of the Translation by H. G. Baynes, 1921.

5. Hammerschlag, Carl A. *The Theft of the Spirit*. New York: Simon & Schuster, 1993, p. 57.

6. "Unconventional Medicine in the United States." *New England Journal of Medicine*, Vol. 328:4, Jan. 28, 1993, pp. 246–252.

7. Glaser, R., and J. Kiecolt-Glaser, eds. *Handbook of Stress and Immunity*. New York: Academic Press, 1994.

8. Kiecolt-Glaser, J., and R. Glaser. "Psychoneuroimmunology: Can Psychological Intervention Modulate Immunity?" *Journal of Consulting and Clinical Psychology*, Vol. 60: 4, 1992, pp. 569–575.

9. Ader, R., D. Felten, and N. Cohen, eds. "Interactions Between the Brain and the Immune System." *Annual Review of Pharmacology and Toxicology*, 30:561–602, 1990.

10. Ader, R., D. Felten, and N. Cohen, eds. *Psychoneuroimmunology*. New York: Academic Press, 1991.

11. Ader, R., and N. Cohen. "Psychoneuroimmunology: Conditioning and Stress." New York: Academic Press, 1991. *Annual Review of Psychology*, 44:53–85, 1993.

12. Bonneau, R. H., J. Kiecolt-Glaser, R. Glaser. "Stress-Induced Modulation of the Immune Response." *Annual of the New York Academy of Science*, 594:253–269, 1990.

13. Locke, Steven, and Douglas Colligan. *The Healer Within: The New Medicine of Mind and Body*. New York: E. P. Dutton, 1986.

14. Sapolsky, Robert M. *Why Zebras Don't Get Ulcers*. New York: Jeremy Tarcher, 1992.

15. Ornstein, R., and C. Senscionis, eds. *The Healing Brain: A Scientific Reader*. New York, London: The Guilford Press, 1990.

16. Byrd, R. C. "Positive Therapeutic Effects of Intercessory Prayer in a Coronary Care Unit Population." *Southern Medical Journal*, Vol. 81(7), July 1988, pp. 826–829.

17. Noen-Hoeksema, S., M. E. P. Seligman, and J. S. Girgus. "Predictors and Consequences of Childhood Depressive Symptoms: A 5-Year Longitudinal Study." *Journal of Abnormal Psychology*, Vol. 101(3), 1992, pp. 405–422.

18. Kamen-Siegel, L., J. Rodin, M. E. P. Seligman, and J. Dwyer. "Explanatory Style and Cell-Mediated Immunity in Elderly Men and Women." *Health Psychology*, 10(4), 1991, pp. 229–235.

19. Langer, E. J., and J. Rodin. "The Effects of Choice and Enhanced Personal Responsibility for the Aged." *Journal of Personality and Social Psychology*, 34:191–198, 1976.

20. Rodin, J. "Aging and Health: Effects of the Sense of Control." *Science*, 233:1271–1276, 1986.

21. Laudenslager, M. L., et al. "Coping and Immunosuppression." *Science*, 221:568–570, 1983.

22. Frankl, Victor. *From Death Camp to Existentialism*. Boston: Beacon Press, 1959. (Reissued as *Man's Search for Meaning*. New York: Simon & Schuster, 1984.)

23. Grunfeld, Dayan I. *The Sabbath*. Jerusalem, New York: Feldheim Publishers, 1954, p. 13.

24. Lusseyran, Jacques. *And There Was Light*. New York: Parabola Books, 1987.

25. Borysenko, John. *Minding the Body, Mending the Mind*. New York: Bantam Books, 1988.

26. Locke, Steven, and Douglas Colligan. *The Healer Within: The New Medicine of Mind and Body*. New York: E. P. Dutton, 1986.

27. *American Medical News*, March 24, 1989.

28. Revicki, Dennis, and Harold May. "Physician Suicide in North Carolina." *Southern Medical Journal*, Vol. 78(10), October 1985, pp. 1205–1207.

29. "Results and Implications of the AMA-APA Physician Mortality Project." *Journal of the American Medical Association*, Vol. 257(21), June 5, 1987, pp. 2949–2953.

30. Dossey, Larry. *Healing Words: The Power of Prayer and the Practice of Medicine*. San Francisco: HarperCollins, 1993, pp. 27.

31. Torah Aura Productions. "Learn Torah With . . ." Com-

mentary on Exodus 6:2–9:35. Vol. 1, No. 14, Dec. 31, 1994, page 1.

Section II—The Ceremonial Seasons: Dawn

—⁓◡⁓—

1. Galinsky, Ellen. *The Six Stages of Parenthood*. Reading, MA: Addison-Wesley, 1987.

2. Klaus, Marshall H., and Kennell, John H. *Bonding: The Beginnings of Parent-Infant Attachment*. St. Louis: C. V. Mosby, 1983.

3. Silverman, H. D. "Role Strain: Illness in a Physician's Family." *Family Systems Medicine*, Vol. 7(4), 1989, pp. 454–457.

4. Kaufman, Barry Neil. "Son-Rise: The Miracle Continues." *Noetic Sciences Review*, 34:22–28, 1995.

5. Bowlby, J. *A Secure Base*. New York: Basic Books, 1988.

6. Ainsworth, M., M. Blehar, E. Waters, and S. Wall. *Patterns of Attachment: A Psychological Study of the Strange Situation*. Hillsdale, NJ: Lawrence Erlbaum, 1978.

7. Hammerschlag, Carl A. *The Theft of the Spirit*. New York: Simon & Schuster, 1993, pp. 116–118.

Section II — The Ceremonial Seasons:
Spring
— ❧ —

1. Erikson, Erik H. *Childhood & Society*. New York: W. W. Norton Co., 1963.

2. Erikson, Erik H. *Identity, Youth and Crisis*. New York: W. W. Norton Co., 1968.

3. Opler, Morris. *An Apache Life Way. The Economic, Social and Religious Institutions of the Chiracahua Indians*. Chicago: University of Chicago Press, 1941.

4. Barrett, S. M. *Geronimo, His Own Story*. New York: E. P. Dutton, 1971.

5. Elkind, David. *All Grown Up and No Place to Go*. Reading, MA: Addison-Wesley, 1984.

6. Duclos, C. W., and S. M. Manson, eds. "Calling from the Rim: Suicidal Behavior Among American Indian and Alaska Native Adolescents." American Indian and Alaska Native Mental Health Research Monograph No. 4. Denver: University Press of Colorado, 1994.

7. Blum, R. W., et al. "American Indian–Alaska Native Youth Health." *The Provider*, August 1992, pp. 137–146.

8. Westlake Van Winkle, N., and P. A. May. "An Update on American Indian Suicide in New Mexico, 1980–1987." *Human Organization*, Vol. 52(3), 1993, pp. 304–315.

9. U.S. National Center for Health Statistics. *Vital Statistics of the United States*. 1990, p. 41.

10. Wolin, S., and L. Bennett. "Family Rituals." *Family Process* Volume 23:403, September 1984.

11. Byrne, Katherine. *A Parent's Guide to Anorexia and Bulimia*. New York: Schocken Books, 1987.

SECTION II—THE CEREMONIAL SEASONS: EARLY SUMMER

1. Levinson, Daniel J. *The Seasons of a Man's Life*. New York: Ballantine Books, 1978.

2. Sheehy, Gail. *Passages*. New York: E. P. Dutton, 1976.

3. Kushner, Lawrence. *The Book of Words*. Woodstock, VT: Jewish Lights Publishing, 1993.

4. Rossi, Ernest L., ed. *The Collected Papers of Milton H. Erickson*. New York: Irvington Publishers, 1980.

5. Haley, Jay. *Uncommon Therapy: The Psychiatric Techniques of Milton H. Erickson, M.D.* New York: W. W. Norton Co., 1973.

6. Rosen, Sidney. *My Voice Will Go With You*. New York: W. W. Norton Co., 1982.

7. Willis, Koko. *Tales of the Night Rainbow*. Honolulu: Rainbow Publishing.

8. Kramer, Peter. *Listening to Prozac*. New York: Viking, 1993.

SECTION II — THE CEREMONIAL SEASONS: LATE SUMMER

1. LeShan, Eda. *The Wonderful Crisis of Middle Age*. New York: David McKay Company, Inc., 1973.
2. Glazer, E. S., and S. L. Cooper. *Without Child*. Lexington, MA: Lexington Books, 1988.

SECTION II — THE CEREMONIAL SEASONS: AUTUMN

1. Jung, Carl Gustav. *Modern Man in Search of a Soul*. p. 57, 1933.
2. Ruebsaat, H., and R. Hull. *The Male Climacteric*. New York: Hawthorne Books, 1975.
3. Sheehy, Gail. *Passages*. New York: E. P. Dutton, 1976.
4. Barbach, Lonnie. *The Pause*. New York: E. P. Dutton, 1993.
5. Sheehy, Gail. *The Silent Passage: Menopause*. New York: Random House, 1992.
6. Greer, Germaine. *The Change*. New York: Alfred Knopf, 1991.

7. "Reveling in Age: Croning Ritual Honors Experience." Tucson: *The Arizona Daily Star*, Nov. 13, 1994.

SECTION II—THE CEREMONIAL SEASONS: EARLY WINTER

1. Schachter-Shalomi, Z., and R. Miller. *From Age-ing to Sage-ing*. New York: Warner Books, 1995.

2. Abrahams, I. *Hebrew Ethical Wills*. Philadelphia: The Jewish Publication Society of America, 1926.

3. Kahn, E., and J. C. Rowe. *Time Dollars*. Emmaus, PA: Rodale Press, 1992.

4. Kohn, Alfie. *The Brighter Side of Human Nature*. New York: Basic Books, 1990.

5. Ornstein, R., and D. Sobel. *Healthy Pleasures*. Reading, MA: Addison-Wesley, 1989.

6. Kiecolt-Glaser, J., and R. Glaser. "Psychoneuroimmunology: Can Psychological Intervention Modulate Immunity?" *Journal of Consulting and Clinical Psychology*, Vol. 60: 4, 1992, pp. 569–575.

7. Landes, K., and D. Umberson. "Social Relationships and Health." *Science* 241:540–545, July 1988.

8. Lynch, James. *The Broken Heart*. New York: Basic Books, 1977.

Section II—The Ceremonial Seasons: Late Winter

1. Dychtwald, Ken. *AgeWave*. Los Angeles: Jeremy Tarcher, 1989.
2. Chopra, Deepak. *Ageless Body, Timeless Mind*. New York: Harmony Books, 1993.

Section II—The Ceremonial Seasons: The Death Transition

1. Einstein, Albert. *What I Believe*. 1930.
2. Hammerschlag, Carl A. *The Dancing Healers*. New York: HarperCollins, 1988, pp. 130–136.
3. Gleick, James. *Genius: The Life and Science of Richard Feynman*. New York: Vintage Books, 1992.
4. Moody, Raymond A. *Life After Life*. New York: Bantam Books, 1975.
5. Moody, Raymond A. *The Light Beyond*. New York: Bantam Books, 1988.

6. Eadie, Betty J. *Embraced by the Light*. Placerville, CA: Gold Leaf Press, 1992.

7. Kubler-Ross, Elizabeth. *On Death and Dying*. New York: MacMillan, 1969.

8. The Support Principle Investigators. *Journal of the American Medical Association*, Vol. 274(20), Nov. 22–29, 1995, pp. 1591–1598.

SECTION III — CREATING PERSONAL RITUALS FOR HEALTH

1. Neihardt, J. G. *Black Elk Speaks*. New York: Washington Square Press, 1959, p. 173.

2. Beck, Renee, and Sydney Barbara Metrick. *The Art of Ritual*. Berkeley, CA: Celestial Arts, 1990.

3. Driver, Tom F. *The Magic of Ritual*. San Francisco: Harper San Francisco, 1991.

4. Achterberg, Jeanne, Barbara Dossey, and Leslie Kolkmeier. *Rituals of Healing*. New York: Bantam Books, 1994.

5. Imber-Black, E., and J. Roberts. *Rituals for Our Times*. New York: HarperCollins, 1993.

6. "Unconventional Medicine in the United States." *New England Journal of Medicine*, Vol. 328 (4), Jan. 28, 1993, pp. 246–252.

7. "Effects of Music on Cardiovascular Reactivity Among

Surgeons." *Journal of the American Medical Association*, Vol. 272(11), Sept. 21, 1994, pp. 882–884.

8. "Music: A Diversionary Therapy." *Today's OR Nurse*, 16(4), July-August, 1994, pp. 17–22.

INDEX

About the Authors

Carl A. Hammerschlag, M.D., is a Yale-trained psychiatrist whose work with Native Americans has been chronicled in his acclaimed book *The Dancing Healers*, which has been adapted by the Public Broadcasting System as its first dramatic miniseries. His second book, *The Theft of the Spirit*, has been endorsed by such distinguished physician-authors as Bernie Siegel. Dr. Hammerschlag is regularly interviewed by radio, television, magazines and newspapers. He is an acclaimed speaker who addresses groups all over the world, as diverse as Fortune 500 companies and the Hopi Tribe. An advisory board member to *Shape Magazine*, he is also a member of the faculty of the University of Arizona College of Medicine and serves on the Board of the Turtle Island Project, a nonprofit educational foundation that has pioneered the use of ritual and ceremony in its programs.

Howard D. Silverman, M.D., is a practicing family physician and Clinical Professor of Family and Community Medicine at the University of Arizona College of Medicine. He started his professional career as a computer scientist, completing graduate studies in artificial intelligence at Massachusetts Institute of Technology. He then completed his medical school training at Stanford University. Dr. Silverman has served as Medical Director of Hospice of the Valley, and as Director of the Family Practice Residency Program at Good Samaritan Regional Medical Center in Phoenix, Arizona. He is currently Medical Director, American Centers for Health and Medicine. He is a founding member of the Turtle Island Project and founding Chairperson of the Group on Spirituality for the Society of Teachers of Family Medicine. He has written and spoken to numerous local and national groups on issues related to medicine, the art of healing, and the integration of spirituality with medical care.